ESSENTIALS IN CYTOPATHOLOGY

Dorothy L. Rosenthal, MD, FIAC, Series Editor

Editorial Board

For further volumes:
http://www.springer.com/series/6996

Liron Pantanowitz
Anil V. Parwani
Editors

Practical Informatics for Cytopathology

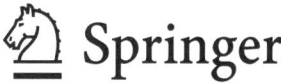 Springer

Editors
Liron Pantanowitz, M.D.
Department of Pathology
University of Pittsburgh
  Medical Center
Pittsburgh, PA, USA

Anil V. Parwani, M.D., Ph.D.,
  M.B.A.
Department of Pathology
University of Pittsburgh
  Medical Center
Pittsburgh, PA, USA

ISSN 1574-9053   ISSN 1574-9061 (electronic)
ISBN 978-1-4614-9580-2   ISBN 978-1-4614-9581-9 (eBook)
DOI 10.1007/978-1-4614-9581-9
Springer New York Heidelberg Dordrecht London

Library of Congress Control Number: 2013957931

Printed on acid-free paper

Springer is part of Springer Science+Business Media (www.springer.com)

To my wife, Heidi, and my children, Joshua and Maya, thanks for your unwavering love and support

Liron Pantanowitz

To Namrata, my wife, and my children, Simran, Varun, and Sanam, who continue to inspire me everyday

Anil V. Parwani

Preface

Pathology informatics has emerged as an essential component of pathology practice, education, and research. Informatics is also critical to help meet current and future challenges. This is not surprising, given that laboratories have become increasingly dependent on computer systems and emerging technology such as digital imaging. Informatics is equally important in the field of cytopathology where it is necessary to support workflow processes, automation, and quality assurance. Current pathology informatics texts cover general topics, but do not deal with issues specific to cytology. Therefore, our goal was to write a book about informatics for cytologists that was practical and relevant to cytopathology. The chapters cover all areas of informatics. We have avoided using distracting technical jargon and provided our readers with tables, boxes, and illustrations for quick and easy reference. This book provides information drawn from our own experience and that of our contributors, who have embraced technology to solve problems and enhance the cytology field.

Pittsburgh, PA, USA   Liron Pantanowitz
                                                        Anil V. Parwani

Acknowledgement

We would like to thank Jacqueline Cuda, Nancy Mauser, Beth Mosley (Kerr), Karen Atkinson, and Dennis J. Wilkinson for helping us review certain sections of this book and for finding the answers to some difficult questions.

Contents

Contributors

Milon Amin, M.D.
Affiliated Pathologists Medical Group, Torrance, CA, USA

R. Marshall Austin, M.D., Ph.D.
Department of Pathology, Magee-Womens Hospital,
University of Pittsburgh Medical Center, Pittsburgh, PA, USA

Ioan C. Cucoranu, M.D.
Department of Pathology, University of Pittsburgh Medical
Center, Pittsburgh, PA, USA

Jacqueline Cuda, B.S., S.C.T. (A.S.C.P).
Department of Pathology, University of Pittsburgh Medical
Center, Pittsburgh, PA, USA

Walid E. Khalbuss, M.D., Ph.D., F.I.A.C.
Department of Pathology, University of Pittsburgh Medical
Center Shadyside, Pittsburgh, PA, USA

Sara E. Monaco, M.D.
Department of Pathology, University of Pittsburgh Medical
Center, Pittsburgh, PA, USA

Liron Pantanowitz, M.D.
Department of Pathology, University of Pittsburgh Medical
Center, Pittsburgh, PA, USA

Seung L. Park, M.D.
Division of Informatics, Department of Pathology, University
of Alabama at Birmingham, Birmingham, AL, USA

Anil V. Parwani, M.D., Ph.D., M.B.A.
Department of Pathology, University of Pittsburgh Medical Center, Pittsburgh, PA, USA

Somak Roy, M.D.
Department of Pathology, University of Pittsburgh Medical Center, Pittsburgh, PA, USA

Muhammad A. Syed, M.D.
Department of Pathology, University of Pittsburgh Medical Center, Pittsburgh, PA, USA

Luke T. Wiehagen, B.S.
Department of Pathology, University of Pittsburgh Medical Center, Pittsburgh, PA, USA

Chapter 1
Introduction to Informatics

Liron Pantanowitz

Clinical (medical) informatics involves the acquisition, storage, use, and management of health care-related data. Informatics in health care not only involves technology but also deals with personnel and the workflow processes impacted by the technology (Fig. 1.1). Informatics applies many principles of computer and information science to clinical practice. It also relies heavily on business, people, and project management skills. Pathology informatics is the practice of informatics specific to pathology (or clinical laboratory) data for clinical service, education, and research. It is different from information technology (IT) and biomedical informatics (or bioinformatics). IT refers more to the technical aspects of this field related to computers, telecommunications (networking), and digital imaging equipment. Biomedical informatics pertains more to biomedical research and clinical or public health care using innovative informatics applications. In practice, pathology informatics involves the application of IT in the laboratory to support and improve clinical workflow, efficiency, and patient care.

L. Pantanowitz, M.D. (✉)
Department of Pathology, University of Pittsburgh Medical Center, Pittsburgh, PA, USA
e-mail: pantanowitzl@upmc.edu

L. Pantanowitz and A.V. Parwani (eds.), *Practical Informatics for Cytopathology*, Essentials in Cytopathology 14, DOI 10.1007/978-1-4614-9581-9_1,

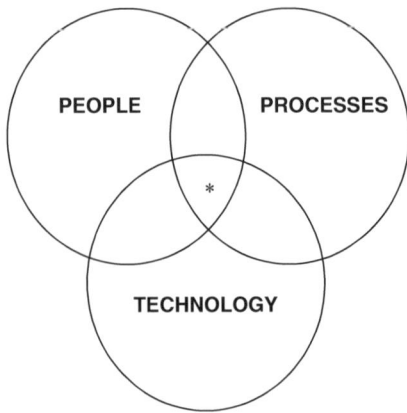

FIG. 1.1 Informatics Venn diagram. The practice of informatics (*asterisk*) involves technology, the people who use, implement, and maintain it, and the workflow processes that are impacted by this technology

With the introduction of regulations and accreditation requirements such as the Clinical Laboratory Improvements Act (CLIA), Health Insurance Portability and Accountability Act (HIPAA), Health Information Technology for Economic and Clinical Health (HITECH) Act, and International Organization for Standardization (ISO), laboratories have begun to pay more attention to compliance and their use of the laboratory information system (LIS) and personal health information (PHI) that belongs to patients. The need for a clinical informatics subspecialty was further precipitated by the ubiquitous use of computers, networking standards such as Health Level Seven (HL7), and the introduction of the electronic medical record (EMR) in the health care environment. Today, there is an Association for Pathology Informatics (API), fellowships available to train in pathology informatics, and a board exam supported by the American Board of Pathology for pathologists to become certified in clinical informatics. Other informatics organizations and resources are listed in Table 1.1.

TABLE 1.1 Clinical informatics resources available on the Internet

Resource	Web address (URL)
American Medical Informatics Association (AMIA)	http://www.amia.org
Association of Medical Directors of Information Systems (AMDIS)	http://www.amdis.org/
Association for Pathology Informatics (API)	http://www.pathologyinformatics.org/
American Telemedicine Association (ATA)	http://www.americantelemed.org/
Digital Pathology Association (DPA)	http://www.digitalpathologyassociation.org/
Healthcare Information and Management Systems Society (HIMSS)	http://www.himss.org/
International Medical Informatics Association (IMIA)	http://www.imia.org/
Journal of Pathology Informatics (JPI)	http://www.jpathologyinformatics.org/
Lab Soft News blog	http://labsoftnews.typepad.com/

Pathologists who deal with informatics are referred to as informaticists (or informaticians). They work closely with lab informatics staff (e.g., LIS manager), IT staff (e.g., chief information officer or CIO, IT analysts), clinical informatics staff (e.g., chief medical information officer or CMIO) and vendors who sell and support information systems. Informaticists play an important role in selecting, implementing and maintaining information systems, middleware and related technology (e.g., digital cameras) in a pathology department. They also serve as change agents between computer programmers and end users. Informatics staff may either work directly for a laboratory (often called LIS staff) or for an institution's IT (or information services) division. In recent years, laboratories have realized the benefit of having pathologists serve as informaticists, since they offer much value with their knowledge of both pathology and informatics.

The practice of cytopathology is increasingly becoming reliant on pathology informatics. This includes the common use of computers (workstations) by cytology staff and those that are attached to or incorporated within lab instruments, as well as the need to work with the LIS and EMR. Cytology staff also need to be informed about medical coding for billing purposes, and understand databases and data mining which play a critical role in their lab's quality management program. More recently, there is a growing demand for automation and efficiency (e.g., barcoding and Lean Six Sigma) in the cytology lab, as well as digital imaging for automated Pap test screening and telecytology. While it is important that cytologists understand the working parts of their light microscopes, it is not essential for them to understand the intricate details of the optics and physics involved in order for them to competently perform their jobs. Similarly, while it is advisable that they have a good working knowledge of informatics in order to successfully practice contemporary cytopathology, cytologists do not necessarily need to have the same technical skills as an IT analyst or computer scientist. This textbook was written to provide the cytologist with a comprehensive overview of the field of pathology informatics. It differs from other informatics books because the content has been specifically tailored and illustrative examples carefully selected for the unique practice of cytopathology.

Chapter 2
Basic Computing

Seung L. Park, Anil V. Parwani, and Liron Pantanowitz

Introduction

Computers have an influential role in our daily professional and personal lives. They are important components of the laboratory information system (LIS), our workstations, and even some lab instruments. They range from large mainframes and racks of servers, to desktop personal computers (PCs) and laptops, as well as small tablets and smartphones. Computers have become increasingly prevalent in medicine, and are important tools for the practice of informatics. Cytologists would be well served to have a general fund of knowledge in the theory and practice behind modern computing.

S.L. Park, M.D. (✉)
Division of Informatics, Department of Pathology,
University of Alabama at Birmingham, Birmingham, AL, USA
e-mail: seungp@uab.edu

A.V. Parwani, M.D., Ph.D., M.B.A. • L. Pantanowitz, M.D.
Department of Pathology, University of Pittsburgh Medical Center,
Pittsburgh, PA, USA
e-mail: parwaniav@upmc.edu; pantanowitzl@upmc.edu

L. Pantanowitz and A.V. Parwani (eds.), *Practical Informatics for Cytopathology*, Essentials in Cytopathology 14, DOI 10.1007/978-1-4614-9581-9_2, © Springer Science+Business Media New York 2014

Binary Data

All computers operate in binary (base-2), i.e., all values are stored as, and all calculations are performed in, zeroes and ones (Table 2.1). This is in contrast to decimal (base-10), which is the standard method of enumerating values that human beings utilize. Hexadecimal (base-16) is often used by programmers because it provides an easily readable, more compact way to visualize and perform operations on binary values.

A bit is a zero (0) or a one (1). A byte is eight bits. Common units of storage are shown in Table 2.2. Note that there are two ways to count units of storage past the byte level—either as powers of 2, or as powers of 10. The reason for this divergence is largely historic. The powers of 10 measurements are now uniformly used by manufacturers of hard drives and other data storage devices. However, many operating systems including Microsoft Windows continue to report storage space in powers of 2, which sometimes gives rise to perceived discrepancies between advertised and actual available storage space.

TABLE 2.1 Binary, decimal, and hexadecimal sample values

Binary	Decimal	Hexadecimal
1	1	0×1
10	2	0×2
1010	10	0×A
10100	20	0×14

TABLE 2.2 Common units of storage

Storage unit	Powers of 10	Powers of 2
Kilobyte (KB)	$10^3 = 1,000$ bytes	$2^{10} = 1,024$ bytes
Megabyte (MB)	$10^6 = 1,000,000$ bytes	$2^{20} = 1,048,576$ bytes
Gigabyte (GB)	$10^9 = 1,000,000,000$ bytes	$2^{30} = 1,073,741,824$ bytes
Terabyte (TB)	$10^{12} = 1,000,000,000,000$ bytes	$2^{40} = 1,099,511,627,776$ bytes

Types of Computers

Different computers have a specific niche in the market. From largest to smallest, the common types of computers include:

- *Mainframes*: These are large, complex, room-spanning computers that boast ultimate stability and predictability, used in mission-critical applications where downtime simply cannot occur (e.g., in the banking industry).
- *Servers*: These high-powered computational platforms can be mounted on standardized frameworks known as racks, either horizontally (the traditional orientation) or vertically (the "blade" orientation). They are seen most often as nodes (connection points) on the Internet, storing and retrieving Web content for users.
- *Workstations*: These are high-powered computational platforms connected to a network, geared toward the act of content creation. Some workstations may be used to input simple data, whereas others may be used for demanding programming or image/video manipulation.
- *Desktop computers*: These are like workstations, but with lower power and usually without specialized peripherals. Such a PC is intended to be used at one location (not portable).
- *Laptop computers*: These portable computers typically have a "clamshell" design in which the screen folds upward on a hinge. They have most of the same components as a desktop computer. They are also called notebooks or netbooks.
- *Tablets*: These are one-piece handheld devices that utilize touch input (touchscreen) as the dominant mode of human–computer interaction. Tablets generally utilize hardware and software derived from smartphones.
- *Smartphones*: These are handheld devices smaller than tablets that utilize touch input as the dominant mode of human–computer interaction. They also integrate a cellular radio for usage as a mobile telephone and internet connectivity device.

Computer Components

A computer can be divided into physical hardware and software. Examples of hardware include the motherboard, disk drive, and keyboard. Additional components (e.g., peripherals) can be connected to the computer such as a monitor, mouse, external hard drive, Webcam, or printer. Examples of software include the operating system (OS), office suites, and Web browsers. The relationship between hardware and software is depicted in Table 2.3.

Hardware

The modern-day computer consists of the following hardware:

- Central processing unit (CPU)
- Motherboard

TABLE 2.3 Relationship between hardware and software[a]

Computer component		Client workstation	Network server
User		Cytopathologist, lab manager, supervisor, cytotechnologist	LIS manager, computer programmer, IT analyst
Software	Applications	LIS, Third-party software	LIS, Database management system
	Operating system	Microsoft, Apple	Unix, Linux, or Other
Hardware		Workstation PC/ Laptop, Mobile devices	Mainframe, Servers

IT information technology, *LIS* laboratory information system, *PC* personal computer

[a]The operating system (OS) is a key component of the system software that manages the hardware resources. Applications (computer programs) employed by users require the OS to function. Similar interactions between hardware and software occur with individual client workstations and servers on a network

- Volatile storage: Registers, cache, and random access memory (RAM)
- Non-volatile storage: Firmware, hard drive, removable disk drives
- Input/output: Graphical processing unit (GPU), human input devices (keyboards, mice, etc.), human output devices (monitors, speakers, etc.), and other peripheral devices

The CPU is considered to be the "brains" of the computer, performing all logical and derived arithmetic operations on binary data. The motherboard is the unit upon which all other components (including the CPU) are mounted and electrically connected (Fig. 2.1). Volatile storage refers to the "working memory" of the computer which is extremely fast. It only holds temporary values and exhibits no permanence. Volatile storage exists in the form of registers and cache built directly into the CPU, as well as random-access memory (RAM) which can be mounted on the motherboard. Non-volatile storage, on the other hand, is slow permanent storage. Such storage consists of firmware (which contains the software that allows the computer to "boot up" and that controls the computer until the OS loads), the hard drive (which is the master permanent storage pool for the rest of the computer), and removable disk drives such as DVD-ROM. Input/output devices provide an interface between humans and computers, as well as an extension of a computer's basic capabilities. Ports (outlets) serve as a physical interface between a computer and peripheral devices (Fig. 2.2). The graphical processing unit (GPU) serves to create images that are displayed on a monitor, which is sometimes also used for general-purpose calculations. Human input devices such as keyboards, mice, and touchscreens allow humans to control the computer. Human output devices such as monitors (or displays) and speakers allow humans to receive signals from the computer.

Software

Common software found on computers includes the OS, user programs, user data, and malware. The OS is so named because it is the central piece of software through which the

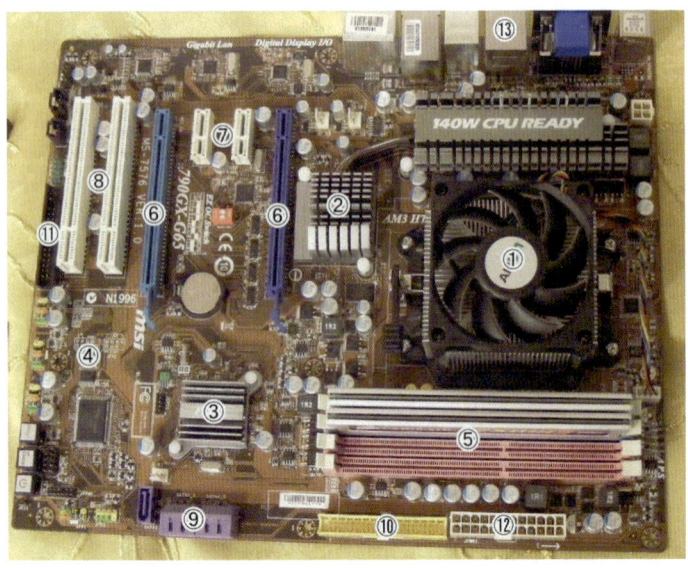

Fig. 2.1 A computer motherboard. (*1*) *CPU*; (2) *northbridge* (controls communication between the CPU and components that require fast access to it, such as video cards); (*3*) *southbridge* (controls communication between the CPU and all other components, such as sound cards); (*4*) *firmware*; (*5*) *RAM slots* (here populated with two sticks of DDR2 SDRAM); (*6*) *PCI-E x16 slot* (for newer video cards); (*7*) *PCI-E x1 slots* (for newer expansion cards); (*8*) *PCI slots* (for expansion cards); (*9*) *SATA ports* (for newer hard drives); (*10*) *IDE port* (for older hard drives); (*11*) *floppy port* (now obsolete); (*12*) *ATX power port*; (*13*) *backplate* (for all other input/output). Photo courtesy of publicphoto.org

capabilities of the computer can be operated. Common operating systems include Microsoft Windows (dominant in desktop computers and in medicine), Mac OS X (found only in Apple computers), Linux (usually seen on servers), Android (found on smartphones and tablets), and iOS (found on Apple handheld devices, including the iPhone and iPad). User programs, also known as applications, are executable packages installed atop the OS and comprise the bulk of what the general public thinks of as "software." These include

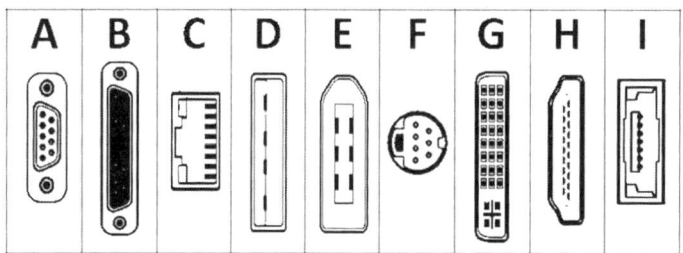

FIG. 2.2 Common ports used to connect cables to a computer. (**a**) Serial port used for serial devices and Personal Digital Assistants (PDAs), (**b**) parallel port used for printers, (**c**) Ethernet/RJ45 used to connect to the Internet and intranet networks at high speed, (**d**) Universal Serial Bus (USB) A, (**e**) Firewire for video cameras and hard drives, (**f**) PS/2 port for mouse or keyboard, as well as S-video for video in/out, (**g**) Digital Video Interface (DVI), (**h**) High-Definition Multimedia Interface (HDMI), and (**i**) eSATA external hard drive port

office suites (e.g., Microsoft Office), Web browsers (e.g., Internet Explorer, Google Chrome), and video games. User programs create, modify, and delete user data which cannot be executed or "run." Malware (e.g., computer viruses and spyware) is defined as any user program that has a harmful effect (intentional or unintentional) on the OS, other user programs, or user data.

Emerging Paradigms in Computing

Web-Based Computing

As Web browsers grew increasingly sophisticated, so too did the webpages they displayed. In the current Internet era, Web pages now have capabilities once only available to installable user programs. This includes online office suites (e.g., Google Docs), online media players (e.g., YouTube), and online social media sites (e.g., Facebook, LinkedIn). This trend is only likely to accelerate in the future.

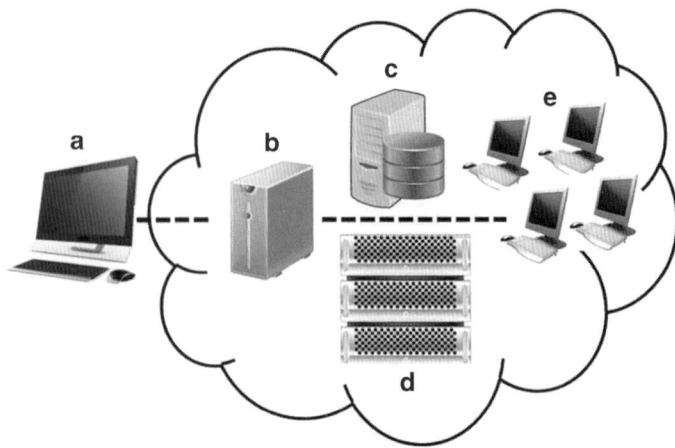

Fɪɢ. 2.3 Schematic of a cloud computing system. On the front end the client's local computer (**a**) connects to the cloud via a control node (**b**). The cloud is comprised of various data storage systems (**c**), application servers (**d**) and a network of other computers (**e**)

Cloud Computing

Cloud computing is used to describe a scenario in which user programs and user data are stored online on distributed servers, to be accessed either via a Web browser or via an install-able application with access to the Internet. It offers end-users computation, software, data access, and storage services without requiring knowledge of the physical location and configuration of the system that delivers such services. In a cloud computing system workload is shifted away from a client's local computer to a network of computers that make up the cloud (Fig. 2.3). The advantage of such a setup is that one can access files anytime, from anywhere, without being teth-ered to a specific computer or location. The disadvantages relate largely to privacy and security, or when Internet con-nectivity is down. With such computing software like a LIS can be offered to laboratories using an Application Service

Provider (ASP) model (also known as Software as a Service or SaaS). The laboratory users in this case access their cloud-based LIS application and all their data stored on a server at a remote location.

Grid Computing

Grid computing is conceptually similar to cloud computing, except that the distributed servers are usually owned by or under the authority of the end user. Grid computing is most often used to bind together many different computer systems to function as a virtual "supercomputer".

Virtualized Computing

This approach is somewhere between traditional desktop computing and cloud computing. In most pathology practices this is how the LIS is deployed, where the LIS is run on a server cluster that the hospital buys, owns and administers. Citrix XenApp (a thin client product that allows users to connect to their corporate applications) is used as a virtualization layer between the server and pathology staff workstations. In other words, the LIS application is not actually installed on the pathology staff computers, but is broadcast through XenApp from the server to their workstations. Virtualized computing is more resource-intensive and places greater strain on the server than cloud computing or traditional desktop computing, but it has several key advantages that make it attractive at this time:

• The Citrix virtualized computing plug-in is available for Windows, Mac OS X, Linux, smartphones, and tablets. This allows applications to be run in a platform-independent fashion on the client side.
• Having centralized data on your own servers means that data ownership is unambiguous, that no third party can see that data, and that you do not have to depend on a third party for server reliability and uptime.

- A large amount of security and encryption is built into Citrix virtualized computing, which means that it is more secure than traditional desktop or cloud computing methods.

Security

Computer security consists of the following layers:

- *Physical security*: Involves (a) making sure that only authorized personnel have physical access to computers, (b) creation of the proper environment (temperature/ humidity controlled) for computer equipment, and (c) provision of proper emergency equipment (e.g., CO_2-based fire extinguishers) in case of emergency.
- *Social security*: This involves hardening one's environment against social engineering attacks, in which the attacker masquerades as a trusted third party in order to gain the trust of the victim.
- *Network security:* Necessitates ensuring that (a) unauthorized network access is prohibited and (b) when such access is detected, the offending device is quarantined and rapidly disconnected before any further security breach can be mounted.
- *Software security*: Requires the usage of appropriately strong passwords and antiviral software.
- *Data security*: Entails the backup of mission-critical data offsite such that even a catastrophic failure will result in minimal loss of data and/or disruption of operations.

Chapter 3
Networking

**Muhammad A. Syed, Anil V. Parwani,
and Liron Pantanowitz**

Introduction

Computer networking refers to the collection of computers connected together via cables or wireless technology. This allows computers to communicate with each other in order to share applications, data, messages, files, resources, and so on. The health care industry relies heavily on computers, and without networking them together it would be extremely challenging to achieve required tasks. Networking in most hospitals is handled by network engineers. While the technical features of networking are beyond the scope of this chapter, a theoretical understanding of key topics is important because of the role they have in today's laboratory information system (LIS).

M.A. Syed, M.D. (✉) • A.V. Parwani, M.D., Ph.D., M.B.A.
L. Pantanowitz, M.D.
Department of Pathology, University of Pittsburgh Medical Center,
Pittsburgh, PA, USA
e-mail: syedma2@upmc.edu; parwaniav@uab.edu;
pantanowitzl@upmc.edu

L. Pantanowitz and A.V. Parwani (eds.), *Practical Informatics
for Cytopathology*, Essentials in Cytopathology 14,
DOI 10.1007/978-1-4614-9581-9_3,
© Springer Science+Business Media New York 2014

Overview of Networks

A computer network is also referred to as a telecommunications network. Devices on networks (e.g., personal computers, hosts, servers) are called nodes. The amount of data that can be transmitted from one point in a network to another in a specified time period (usually seconds) is known as data bandwidth. "Broadband" refers to extensive bandwidth features of a transmission medium, and its ability to transfer multiple signals simultaneously. Pathology laboratories typically depend on two types of networks, including:

- *Intranet*: A private computer network that uses Internet technology to securely share information and/or computing services within an organization.
- *Internet*: A global public system of interconnected computer networks that use the standard Internet protocol suite (see section in Chap. 3 "Protocols and Standards").

Various network topologies (physical layout of connected devices) are typically used in combination to build a network. Some basic topologies include Bus, Ring, Star, Mesh and Tree network structures.

Network Types

Networks can also be categorized by their range (i.e., how far they are connected), scale, type of connection (wired and/or wireless), and purpose. Common examples include:

- *Local area network (LAN)*: This type of network is geographically limited (e.g., a network confined to a medical center).
- *Wide area network (WAN)*: These networks cover a much larger geographic area, and typically connect two or more LANs (e.g., a network across a city).

- *Personal area network (PAN)*: This type of network is used to connect an individual's computer with nearby devices (e.g., printer). Wireless technology (e.g., Bluetooth) works well with such a short-range network.
- *Virtual private network (VPN)*: These networks allow users to work over a public network (Internet) while maintaining security and privacy. They employ technology to accomplish this, such as tunneling protocols (e.g., L2TP), which separates private and general network traffic.
- *Storage area network (SAN)*: These networks are dedicated to storing data. They make storage devices (e.g., disk arrays) accessible to computers and servers.

Network Architecture

Network architecture takes into account several features including the physical layout of the network, functional relationship among devices on the network, and technology (e.g., communication protocols). The client–server and peer-to-peer models are the ones most widely used today (Fig. 3.1).

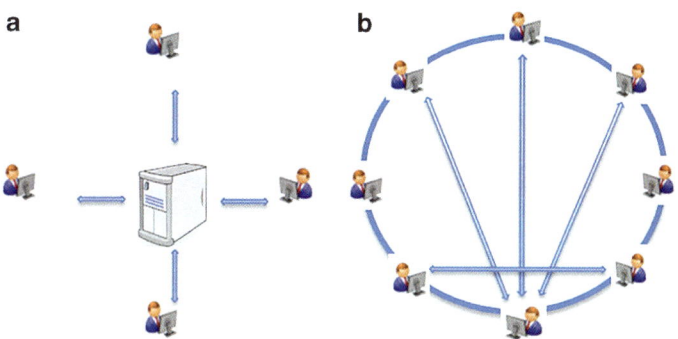

FIG. 3.1 (**a**) A network configuration in a client–server model. (**b**) Network of a peer-to-peer system of computers without a central server

Client–Server Model

There are two components in a client–server model: client workstations (spread throughout the network), and a central server (usually a powerful host computer). The server receives requests from networked clients. The client's workstation in turn displays the result the server returns. Many clients can access the server simultaneously. For instance, in a hospital environment when a client in the emergency department enters information about a patient in their workstation, this information gets stored in a permanent database on a server. When the hospital's pathology laboratory receives a specimen from this patient, they can now access this information from the server. One advantage of running a client–server model is that only the data on the server requires back-up, for data safety in the event of a server failure. These networks can be further set up with/without applications and resources installed on the client's workstation. This will depend on whether they are thin, thick or smart clients.

Thin Client

On a thin client workstation, limited processing of information can be accomplished with fewer applications. That is because the function of a thin client is primarily data entry. The advantage of having thin clients on a network includes easy maintenance and reduced cost. However, the thin client depends heavily on the server's applications, which is a problem when it fails. A "dumb terminal" refers to a workstation that consists of just a monitor with a keyboard and mouse, connected to the server over the network, with no processing ability.

Thick Client

A thick client refers to a computer on a network that can process the user's request by using a set of locally installed applications. The need to access the server is minimal, and reserved largely to authentication or some archiving of data. Processing high bandwidth tasks locally and not off the server significantly reduces network traffic. However, this model requires local installation of multiple applications and increased hardware to support processing. In addition, individual upgrades are more difficult to maintain and at a much higher cost.

Smart Client

In recent years, the trend is shifting towards a newer Web-based architecture. This model combines the benefit of thin and thick clients. In this model the client represents a computer connected to the Internet that accesses server applications using Web services. These Web applications (even an entire LIS) can have the look and feel of actual desktop applications. No installation is required and updates can occur automatically without user action. Smart clients are capable of working with data "offline," i.e., even when an Internet connection is not available. "Rich Internet Applications" (RIA) used to support this network model include Flash and Java applets. An applet (or plug-in) is a small application that performs a specific task that runs within a larger program.

Peer-to-Peer (P2P) Model

In a P2P network (also called a decentralized or distributed network) all computers (called "peers") on the network equally use and share responsibilities for data processing. They all simultaneously function as both "clients" and "servers" to the other nodes on the network. For example, an application installed on one computer can be accessed from any machine on the network. This type of network is ideal for small LANs (e.g., interconnected computers situated physically near each other), is inexpensive and easy to maintain. However, the downside is compromised security.

Interfaces

In the health care environment, disparate information systems and devices usually do not readily link to each other (i.e., they do not just "plug and play"). Rather, they rely on an interface created by a blend of software (e.g., codes) and hardware (e.g., plugs and sockets) that allows devices on a network to communicate and exchange data. A program that integrates and centralizes many different application interfaces is known as an interface engine. Several interfaces are found in the pathology lab, including:

- *Admission/Discharge/Transfer (ADT) interface*: This interface is responsible for electronic feeds containing patient demographic data from a hospital information system (HIS) into the LIS.
- *Order entry (OE) interface*: This interface transmits a health care provider's order for a lab test (selected from a test menu), placed in a clinical information system, to the LIS.
- *Result entry interface*: This interface transmits results from the LIS to the electronic medical record (EMR) system.
- *Billing interface*: This interface is used to send financial data (e.g., insurance information, fee codes associated with diagnoses) from the LIS to either a hospital billing system or third party vendor for billing and reimbursement.
- *Instrument interface*: A link between an information system (e.g., LIS) and its hardware instruments (e.g., autostainer).

Protocols and Standards

A protocol is a set of rules used to exchange information over a network. Based on the Open Systems Interconnection (OSI) model a protocol is divided into seven layers (Table 3.1). Each layer is responsible for a different

TABLE 3.1 The seven layers of the OSI model

Layer	Key function
Application layer	Displays data and images in a format that humans can comprehend (user interface)
Presentation layer	Converts data from a standards-based format to one that is understandable by a local device
Session layer	Keeps track of file transfer requests, Web page retrievals and unique sessions with remote servers
Transport layer	Recovers lost or damaged data from an error
Network layer	Facilitates routing of data by embedding and mapping the source and delivery destinations into data packets
Data link layer	Checks for errors that may have occurred with transmission and packages data to be forwarded
Physical layer	Handles the raw data which travels to and from the receiving and sending device

part of the communication process. Although there are many communication protocols, the protocol most useful for cytologists is the Internet Protocol suite. This protocol, also called the Transmission Control Protocol/Internet Protocol (TCP/IP), is the foundation of the Internet. Web browsers use TCP/IP to communicate with Web servers.

Health Level 7 (HL7)

HL7 is the standard used for exchanging information between health care applications. The benefit of having everyone use the same HL7 standard is that it promotes interoperability. The format in HL7 consists of multiple segments. Each segment, in turn, is delimited with fields (Fig. 3.2). A translation table may still be needed for cross-reference between different systems and their HL7 codes.

```
001   MSH|^~\&|HIS|BA6|AP-LIS||2013080311700|SMS

002   EVN|A04A|2013080311700

003   PID|0123|5432^UPMC||CYTOFNA||F||W|1025|4125551212|ETC

004   PV|0001|OP|CYTOLOGY^^|R|||FNAMSTER^RAD||ETC

005   DG|0001||CYTO||

006   GT|0001||CYTOFNA|1025|4125551212||NOCHARGE|ETC

007   IN||0678945|UPMCHEALTHPLAN
```

FIG. 3.2 An example of an inbound HL7 message being transmitted from a Hospital Information System (HIS) to the Anatomic Pathology LIS (AP-LIS). Segments include *MSH* message header, *EVN* event, *PID* patient identification, *PV* patient visit details, *GT* guarantor, *INS* insurance

Network Security

Security is important to protect a network from threats and unauthorized activities. There are many threats on the Internet such as viruses, spyware, worms, hackers, and identity theft. This poses a serious problem for hospitals and laboratories that need to connect to the Internet. Firewalls are one way to help mitigate such threats. Firewalls are typically installed at the entry/exit point of a network, allowing authorized users access to network recourses while blocking illegal intrusion (Fig. 3.3). Firewalls check network packets of data for their authenticity, to determine if they are coming from a previously identified source such as a trusted IP address or a domain. A Denial-of-Service (DoS) attack is an attempt to render a host/server or network resource unavailable to its intended users by over-burdening it with a very high number of requests. Recent advances in networking like packet filtering have reduced the impact of DoS attacks. Another security measure is to employ encryption, which is the alteration of sensitive data into a cipher text that is no longer in a readable format. Once the encrypted data reaches its intended destination, a decryption key is required to recover and read the data.

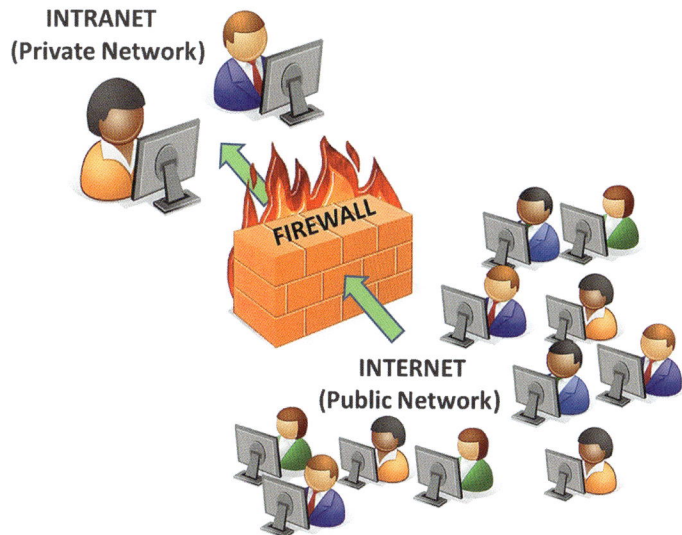

Fɪɢ. 3.3 A firewall is designed to protect a private network from the Internet

Chapter 4
Databases

Seung L. Park, Anil V. Parwani, and Liron Pantanowitz

Introduction

Databases are organized collections of digital data. They are created and manipulated by programs known as database management systems (DBMS), many of which are designed for very specific purposes (e.g., Microsoft Excel, Microsoft Access, MySQL, Oracle). Databases are of intrinsic interest to cytologists because they are used not only to organize data in the laboratory information system (LIS), but also to deal with data for quality assurance (QA) purposes, business intelligence and research.

S.L. Park, M.D. (✉)
Division of Informatics, Department of Pathology,
University of Alabama at Birmingham,
Birmingham, AL, USA
e-mail: seungp@uab.edu

A.V. Parwani, M.D., Ph.D., M.B.A. • L. Pantanowitz, M.D.
Department of Pathology, University of Pittsburgh Medical Center,
Pittsburgh, PA, USA
e-mail: parwaniav@uab.edu; pantanowitzl@upmc.edu

L. Pantanowitz and A.V. Parwani (eds.), *Practical Informatics for Cytopathology*, Essentials in Cytopathology 14, DOI 10.1007/978-1-4614-9581-9_4,
© Springer Science+Business Media New York 2014

Database Fundamentals

There are certain basic functionality requirements that all databases, no matter what their intended purpose, must satisfy—they are to Create, Read, Update, and Delete (CRUD) data. Consider the following example with a laboratory information system (LIS):

- Without the ability to *create* new accession numbers, there would be no way to enter specimens into the system.
- Without the ability to *read* already-existing cases, there would be no way to report signed-out cases.
- Without the ability to *update* cases, there would be no way to correct errors in reports or to add an addendum when necessary.
- Without the ability to *delete*, old terminology or test protocols that are no longer valid could never be removed from the system.

Atomicity, consistency, isolation, and durability (ACID) are important criteria to ensure that databases are reliable at all times.

- *Atomicity* requires database modifications to be "all or nothing," as no partial transactions are allowed.
- *Consistency* requires that only valid data be written to the DBMS.
- *Isolation* requires that only one user at a time can access or modify a given record.
- *Durability* requires that the DBMS is able to recover a committed transaction if there is a system failure.

Database Models

Every database is defined by its model, which specifies what the database can and cannot do. There are many models, some of which are obsolete. Table 4.1 summarizes the most popular database models. The flat, hierarchical and relational models are the most prevalent in laboratory information systems, and will therefore be further discussed.

TABLE 4.1 Common database models

Model	Description	Advantages	Disadvantages	Examples
Flat	The simplest and most common kind of database model. Consists of a single two-dimensional table of elements.	Simple Intuitive Widely available Easily imported into other models	Not robust For single-user only Unwieldy when large Duplication of data	Spreadsheet Comma-separated values (CSV) Tab-separated values (TSV)
Hierarchical	Navigational in style. Data is organized in a tree structure (with "parent" and "child" nodes).	Simple Intuitive Efficient at describing nested and sorted data	Inefficient with many common database operations Low-level and inflexible Lower productivity than relational model databases	IBM Information Management System (IMS) Microsoft Windows Registry All XML databases
Network	Navigational in style. Similar to the hierarchical model, except that each node can have multiple "parents" and "children." Works similar to computer network topologies.	Intuitive Flexible Extremely fast record retrieval	Low-level Database loading and node reorganization can be slow Lower productivity than relational model databases	DEC VAX DBMS RDM Embedded Object-oriented databases

(continued)

TABLE 4.1 (continued)

Model	Description	Advantages	Disadvantages	Examples
Relational	The dominant database model in use today. A mathematical model defined by set theory. Similar to the flat model, except that it has multiple tables that can be linked to each other by way of key values. Uses a standardized syntax called Structured Query Language (SQL).	Ubiquitous Freely available Standardized by SQL Can be accessed with popular programming languages by way of extensions	Higher system requirements than hierarchical and network model databases Joining operations (associating data) are essential, which are complex and computationally expensive	IBM DB2 mySQL PostgreSQL SQLite HSQLDB Oracle Database Microsoft SQL server
Object-oriented	Uses object structures that can be directly used in low- and high-level object-oriented programming languages.	Intuitive to programmers High-performance Works well for distributed architectures	Standardized through the Object Database Management Group (ODMG) Poor interoperability	Objectivity/DB MUMPS implementations
Document-oriented	A higher-level approach that emphasizes documents over structured tables. Records can have a nonstandard amount of information, and need not have the same fields.	Intuitive to nonprogrammers Simple enough not to use SQL	Not standardized Not always of high-performance Usually do not use SQL	Lotus Notes CouchDB Apache Jackrabbit RavenDB All XML databases

eXtensible Markup Language (XML)	A hierarchical markup language that allows for documents to be encoded in machine-readable form. Each XML document is defined by its "schema," which is a templated hierarchy that can be created by the end user.	Intuitive to users familiar with other markup languages, most notably Hypertext Markup Language (HTML) XML documents are machine- and human-readable, and do not require specialized tools Ubiquitous and "made for" the Web Used by standards bodies including Health Level 7 (HL7)	Sacrifices performance for readability Has disadvantages of earlier hierarchical model databases Impossible to truly standardize, as anyone can write their own schema Multiple competing syntaxes	BaseX Oracle Berkeley DB eXist MarkLogic Server
Graph	Based on graph theory. Made up of nodes which are connected to one another by "edges" that represent node-to-node relationships. Each node has intrinsic "properties." Edges and properties can be arbitrarily defined, and need not be codified in tables.	Scalable for large data sets Very flexible Intuitive to object-oriented programmers Can be high-performance Good for queries commonly used in biomedical research	Not fast at performing the same operation on large numbers of data elements Not standardized Fewer user tools than relational DBMS	AllegroGraph Cytoscape Neo4j OrientDB VertexDB

(continued)

TABLE 4.1 (continued)

Model	Description	Advantages	Disadvantages	Examples
Entity-Attribute-Value	A sparse-matrix model where each entity might potentially have a vast number of attributes, but the number of attributes actually applying to a given entity is a small subset. Stores only nonempty values. Relies heavily on metadata systems to provide meaningful relationships across the database. Implemented on top of a relational DBMS.	Intuitive to clinical datasets. Can be manipulated through SQL. Good for distributed cloud-based data stores	Reliance on metadata means that the way data are stored and retrieved is completely decoupled from the way they need to be presented. Since they are implemented on top of a relational DBMS, they have similar limitations and bottlenecks	Cerner Millenium (some portions) Amazon EC2 SimpleDB Microsoft Windows Azure Table Storage Google App Engine
Dimensional	Consists of multidimensional cubes. Almost all business intelligence and data mining software use this model.	Can be manipulated through SQL. Good for multidimensional data mining and analysis. Good at illustrating trends and defining endpoints	Extremely complex. Computationally expensive. Require constant background joins and pivot table style operations, which create bottlenecks in performance. Nonintuitive if not versed in database programming	IBM Cognos Business Intelligence Altosoft Insight SAS Business Analytics Jaspersoft Business Intelligence Informix MetaCube SAP Crystal Reports

Flat Database Model

This is the simplest database model and most ubiquitous in daily life. Every single time someone produces a table with columns and rows of data they create a flat database file. This construct is surprisingly powerful and frequently employed in presenting cytology data for QA purposes (see Table 9.2 as an example in Chap. 9). Success with this type of database is dependent on how well the user organized their data. They also suffer from many data inconsistency problems, and become increasingly unwieldy as the dataset becomes large and/or more complex. Modern electronic medical records do not utilize the flat model.

Hierarchical Database Model

This database model, previously thought to be obsolete, is in use again with eXtensible Markup Language (XML). In the hierarchical model, data are represented in a tree-like structure where information is represented using parent/child relationships. Each "parent" can have many "children," but each "child" has only one "parent" (one-to-many relationship). This gives rise to a highly nested data structure, which is ideal for the description of structured text documents (Fig. 4.1). This structure is very computationally efficient, but can be difficult for human beings to manipulate. Electronic medical records that utilize the hierarchical model include Epic, VistA/CPRS, and Misys/Sunquest.

Relational Database Model

This is currently the dominant model used in laboratory information systems and electronic medical records. This model trades performance for productivity. It is best characterized as a dataset consisting of multiple related 2-dimen-

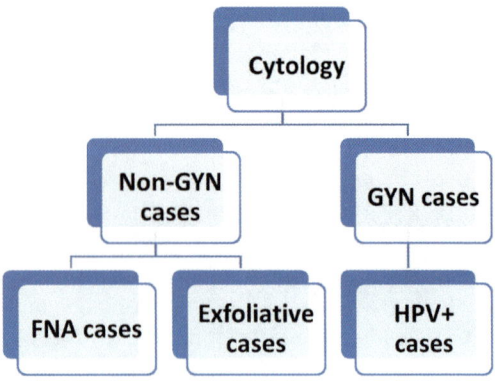

FIG. 4.1 Example of a hierarchical database model

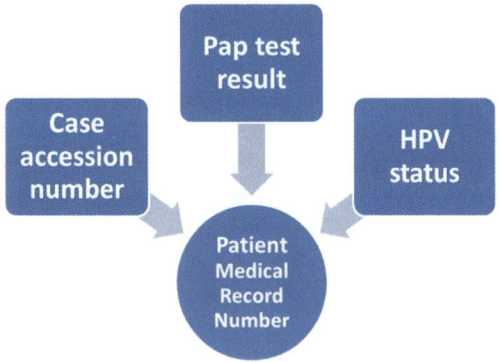

FIG. 4.2 Example of a relational database model. The key value linking the tables (so-called relations) in this diagram is the patient medical record number common to each dataset

sional tables, each of which can link into others through key values (an entry in a specific column and row/tuple) (Fig. 4.2). There are special ways of organizing tables (called normalization) in the relational model to avoid data redundancy. These datasets have a standard interface for CRUD known as

Structured Query Language (SQL). Electronic medical records that utilize the relational model include Cerner Millenium, Orchard Path, and OpenEMR.

Data Warehouses

In data warehousing, data are continually extracted from production sources, copied, cleaned, transformed, catalogued, and made available for purposes such as data mining and decision support. Data warehouses are attractive because they:

- Maintain data history even if the production sources do not
- Integrate data from multiple source systems that may be mutually compatible with one another, providing a central enterprise-wide view
- Eliminate inconsistency and anomaly in enterprise data by applying a consistent code and metadata model
- Allow for complex, processor-intensive decision support systems to be run without affecting the production environment
- Allow for processor-intensive data mining and online analytic processing to be run, again without affecting the production environment

Data warehouses are primarily used for a broad class of computer analytic techniques called "business intelligence." The overarching aim of these technologies is to support better decision making, and to attempt to make sense of the vast amount of data that flows through any given organization (Fig. 4.3).

Data Mining

Data mining refers to the act of having a computer automatically analyze large quantities of data to identify meaningful, statistically significant patterns. With algorithmic advances in

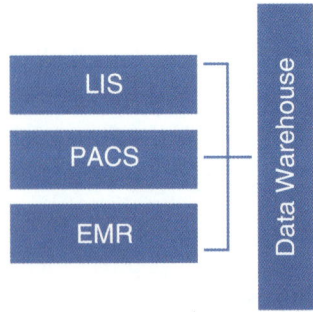

FIG. 4.3 Data warehouse overview. The data vault (central repository) of the warehouse in this example is created by integrating data
uploaded from several disparate operational information systems
including a laboratory information system (LIS), radiology picture
archiving and communication system (PACS), and electronic medical record (EMR)

computer science like neural networks, genetic algorithms and
support vector machines, data mining has become increasingly
sophisticated. Large-scale bioinformatics research projects
and clinical trials often depend on mining large sets of data.
Such analyses together with digital visualization of the findings can be computationally very demanding.

Chapter 5
Coding

Seung L. Park, Jacqueline Cuda, and Liron Pantanowitz

Introduction

In practice, the use of appropriate codes is important for proper handling, accessioning, reporting, and billing of cytology cases. Coding systems are mechanisms to represent a set of related real-world concepts using defined codes or terms that can be utilized by data processing systems. They range in complexity from straightforward lists of concepts to complex multi-axial, hierarchical codes (Table 5.1). Coding systems employ a controlled terminology (Table 5.2), which is a finite

S.L. Park, M.D. (✉)
Division of Informatics, Department of Pathology,
University of Alabama at Birmingham, Birmingham, AL, USA
e-mail: seungp@uab.edu

J. Cuda, B.S., S.C.T. (A.S.C.P.) • L. Pantanowitz, M.D.
Department of Pathology, University of Pittsburgh Medical Center,
Pittsburgh, PA, USA
e-mail: cudajm@upmc.edu; pantanowitzl@uab.edu

L. Pantanowitz and A.V. Parwani (eds.), *Practical Informatics for Cytopathology*, Essentials in Cytopathology 14,
DOI 10.1007/978-1-4614-9581-9_5,
© Springer Science+Business Media New York 2014

TABLE 5.1 Different coding systems

Code	Definition	Key purpose
CPT	Current procedural terminology	Listing of medical procedures and services performed by health care providers, utilized in electronic billing transactions
ICD	International classification of diseases	Terms devoted to describing medical conditions, often used in electronic billing transactions
LOINC	Logical observations identifiers and codes	A database and universal standard for identifying medical laboratory observations
SNOMED	Systematized nomenclature of medicine	A collection of medical terms that provides a consistent way to index, store, retrieve, and aggregate medical data across specialties and sites of care

set of terms with an agreed-upon meaning that allows users to confidently communicate information to a receiver who will be able to interpret the message unambiguously. Many coding systems were developed to allow automation of administrative functions, such as billing. To bill for a test, a cytology laboratory will need to submit a claim that includes the International Classification of Diseases (ICD) code which justifies medical necessity, and a Current Procedural Terminology (CPT) code which describes what was performed. Codes facilitate electronic capture and recall of standardized data for other purposes as well, such as epidemiologic research, monitoring health care utilization, and quality improvement activities.

Common Coding Systems

International Classification of Diseases (ICD)

The International Classification of Diseases, first formulated in 1893, is a family of classification systems with many variants. The most widely used version in the USA is currently

TABLE 5.2 Key terms used in coding systems

Term	Explanation
Concept	A fundamental unit of meaning within a terminology or a classification system (e.g., an anatomic structure)
Term	A word or phrase that names a particular concept; there may be multiple terms which convey the identical concept (e.g., "stroke" = "cerebrovascular accident")
Classification	A system for organizing concepts within a particular area of knowledge into related groupings; based on a previously defined system of relationships (e.g., ICD, which organizes many of the concepts by anatomic location or function)
Terminologies	Also known as nomenclatures, these are sets of terms for concepts in a particular area of knowledge
Vocabulary	A specialized form of nomenclature that additionally provides definitions for terms (e.g., ICD, which is both a terminology and a classification, but not a vocabulary)
Ontology	A vocabulary which includes information about the relationships between concepts; this allows for an understanding of the structure of the information, and facilitates advanced information processing
Semantic relationships	These are expressions of the connections between various concepts (e.g., the fact that human papillomavirus is a virus, and also a causative agent of certain diseases)
Axes	These are hierarchies in which linked concepts with shared attributes (e.g., names, values) are arranged (grouped)

ICD-9-CM (CM = clinical modification), which is being replaced by ICD-10-CM. Development of ICD-11 is currently underway. ICD-9-CM was implemented to provide a system for classifying morbidity data and assigning codes to diagnoses and procedures associated with hospital utilization. The National Center for Health Statistics (NCHS) and Centers for Medicare/Medicaid Services (CMS) are responsible for

TABLE 5.3 Comparison between ICD-9 and ICD-10 codes

ICD-9	ICD-10
Limited space for adding new codes	More flexible for adding new codes
Codes are 3–5 characters in length	Codes can be 3–7 characters in length
First digit may be alpha or numeric, and digits 2–5 are numeric	Digit 1 is alpha, digits 2 and 3 are numeric, and digits 4–7 may be alpha or numeric
Codes have limited detail	Very specific codes
Codes lack laterality	Includes laterality (i.e., codes identifying right versus left)

overseeing changes and modifications to ICD-9-CM. Structurally, ICD-9-CM is composed of three volumes: volume 1: tabular list of diseases and injuries; volume 2: alphabetic index to diseases; volume 3: procedure testing. Valid codes in ICD-9-CM range between three and five digits: three digits to the left of a decimal point, and up to two digits to the right. As the number of digits increases, so too does the specificity of the code: for instance, 180 is the ICD-9-CM code for "malignant neoplasm of cervix uteri", whereas 180.1 is the ICD-9-CM code for "malignant neoplasm of exocervix". ICD-9-CM has been very useful for over 20 years, but the ability to add new codes is relatively limited. ICD-10 allows for more codes and permits tracking of many new diagnoses and procedures (Table 5.3). ICD-10-CM is used for diagnosis codes and intended to replace volumes 1 and 2. ICD-10-PCS is for procedure codes and intended to replace volume 3. With ICD-10 the codes can be up to seven characters long, with three characters to the left of the decimal point indicating the category and three characters to the right of the decimal point indicating level of detail. For Pap tests, primary ICD codes are provided by the referring physician. For non-gynecologic cytology specimens, ICD codes are assigned by the pathologist based on their diagnosis (unless the diagnosis is nonspecific; then a relevant clinician provided ICD code should be used).

Current Procedural Terminology (CPT)

CPT, now in its fourth edition, is a set of codes and descriptive terms published by the American Medical Association (AMA) and used for reporting medical services performed by physicians. It occupies a key role in the flow of billing and claims information in the USA. It is essential in order to ensure that you have correctly represented the work performed on a given specimen and to ensure that you received the proper payment for these services. Using CPT codes to bill for clinical lab services is typically straightforward, but the unique structure of cytopathology service codes implies that there are a number of instances where interpretation may be needed. CPT has been adopted by the Centers for Medicare and Medicaid Services (CMS) as part of the Healthcare Common Procedure Coding System (HCPCS) and has been mandated for use in a variety of billing and reporting systems throughout the USA. CPT and HCPCS are the procedure code set for electronic transactions related to physician services, laboratory testing, and a variety of other services and procedures as mandated by the Health Insurance Portability and Accountability Act of 1996 (HIPAA).

CPT codes for the pathology laboratory typically fall between 80000 and 89999. There are hundreds of codes for clinical laboratory testing, but only a few for cytopathology (Table 5.4). For diagnostic Pap tests, CPT codes are used exclusively (Table 5.5). These CPT codes are derived from information provided by the clinician. HCPCS codes are used for screening Pap tests. It is important to be aware that only a referring physician can classify a Pap test as screening, high risk or diagnostic. CPT codes assigned to Pap tests are also based upon whether the specimen involves a conventional smear or liquid based preparation, if there was manual and/or computer-assisted screening performed, and if a pathologist was involved with interpretation. CPT codes for nongynecological cytology cases vary based on the sample preparation requirements (Table 5.4). In order to use the immediate evaluation code 88172, the patient must still be

TABLE 5.4 Common cytology CPT codes

CPT code	Description
Gynecologic cytopathology	
88141	Pap test requiring pathologist review (professional component for all Pap tests)
88142	Manual screening under pathologist supervision (technical component for liquid-based Pap tests)
88164	Manual screening under pathologist supervision (technical component for conventional Pap tests)
88174	Manual screening and computer re-screen (equivalent to automated screening of ThinPrep Pap tests and no further review for Focal Point)
88175	Liquid based Pap test with screening by an automated system
P3000	Conventional Pap smear with no pathologist review
P3001	Conventional Pap smear requiring pathologist review
G0123	Liquid based Pap test with no pathologist review
G0144	Liquid based Pap test that is automated
G0145	Liquid based Pap test that is automated with manual re-screening
Non-gynecologic cytopathology	
88104	Fluid requiring simple smear preparation
88108	Fluid requiring concentration technique (e.g., cytospin)
88112	Fluid requiring thin layer preparation
88160	Smear(s) prepared by client
88161	Smear(s) requiring preparation
88162	Multiple smears (five or more) requiring extended study
88172	Determination of adequacy of specimen
88173	FNA interpretation
88177	Additional FNA evaluation episodes
88305	Fluid requiring cell block preparation

TABLE 5.5 Definition of screening and diagnostic Pap tests

Screening (routine) Pap tests

   No current sign/symptoms related to the cervix

   No previous abnormal Pap test

   No high risk factors for cervical cancer

Screening (high risk) Pap tests

   Early onset of sexual activity

   Multiple sexual partners

   History of sexually transmitted disease

   Less than three negative Pap tests in 7 years

   Daughter of a mother given DES

   Abnormal Pap test in the last 3 years

Diagnostic Pap tests

   Previously diagnosed cancer of the vagina, cervix, or uterus

   Previous abnormal Pap test

   Current abnormal finding of the vagina, cervix, uterus, or adnexae

   Significant complaint referable to the female genital tract

   Any sign/symptom that might be related to a gynecologic disorder

present in order to obtain more FNA passes if deemed necessary. There are also a variety of codes for additional studies that may be ordered at the discretion of the pathologist, such as 88312 for special stains to detect microorganisms, 88313 for histochemical stains, and 88342 for immunohistochemical stains. Sometimes it can be difficult to accurately determine which CPT codes to use. To illustrate this point, examples of different cytology scenarios are shown in Table 5.6. Most routine surgical pathology specimens fall into one of six levels of service, which are arranged in accordance with the level of effort required for a typical case of a given type. For example, an incidental appendix is a level II (CPT code 88302) whereas a colectomy for tumor is a level VI (88309).

TABLE 5.6 Examples illustrating the use of CPT codes for cytology

Scenario 1

A pleural fluid obtained by a clinician via thoracentesis is submitted directly to the cytology laboratory. The cytotechnologist prepares one ThinPrep, two cytospins, and one cell block. The cytopathologist does not order ancillary studies. The final cytopathology reports is as follows:

PLEURAL FLUID, RIGHT, THORACENTESIS:

    A. SATISFACTORY FOR INTERPRETATION.

    B. NEGATIVE FOR MALIGNANT CELLS.

    C. REACTIVE MESOTHELIAL CELLS.

The correct CPT codes assigned to this case are 88108 (for the cytospin), 88112 (for the ThinPrep), and 88305 (for the cell block). However, as only one concentration method can be billed, the proper coding on this case will be 88112 and 88305 only.

Scenario 2

A CT-guided FNA of a lung mass is performed by the radiologist in three passes and evaluated on-site by a cytopathologist. Six direct smears, one cell block, and five immunohistochemical stains are prepared. The final cytopathology report is as follows:

LUNG, LEFT UPPER LOBE, CT-GUIDED FINE NEEDLE ASPIRATION:

    A. SATISFACTORY FOR INTERPRETATION.

    B. POSITIVE FOR MALIGNANT CELLS.

    C. NON-SMALL-CELL CARCINOMA.

The correct CPT codes assigned to this case are 88173 (FNA interpretation and report), 88172 (immediate study for adequacy assessment), 88305 (for a cell block), and 88342 ×5 (for immunohistochemical stains).

Logical Observations Identifiers and Codes (LOINC)

LOINC is a coding system to ensure that when two different parties (physicians or laboratories) talk about a test result, the individual results can be uniquely and unambiguously specified. LOINC was first developed in 1995 by the Regenstrief Institute and Indiana University. It was created to address the issue that even though electronic communication of laboratory results was being accomplished using standardized messaging systems, the codes used to identify results were usually local codes, as there was no universal standard. The scope of LOINC is broader than just clinical laboratory results, although the majority of codes are indeed laboratory-related. There are currently close to 70,000 codes in LOINC, with more codes being added on a daily basis. Code numbers are assigned as entries are developed and currently consist of up to five numeric digits followed by a hyphen and a check digit to detect errors. Unlike other coding systems, LOINC observes no inherent organization of codes: for instance, 50872-1 denotes a lithium analysis on hair, whereas the next code in sequence 50873-9 denotes a magnesium–creatinine ratio in a 24 h sample. Each LOINC code maps to specific points in up to six different fields or axes (Tables 5.7 and 5.8). While LOINC codes cover almost all common laboratory analytes, and a variety of other observations (e.g., Gleason score), there is certain information that is not included in LOINC (e.g., particular assay methods and specific sampling locations). LOINC is concerned with specifying the clinical question being asked and not necessarily the answers to those questions. LOINC can, for instance, be used to code the observation that bacteria were identified by culture, but the identity of those bacteria must be coded in a totally different system (e.g., ICD-9-CM). Most large laboratories have incorporated LOINC within their electronic result messages. This is beneficial, because LOINC can improve communication across networks between different information systems.

Systematized Nomenclature of Medicine (SNOMED)

SNOMED began in 1965 as a Systematized Nomenclature of Pathology (SNOP). It was subsequently further developed, with the creation of SNOMED Clinical Terms (SNOMED-CT)

TABLE 5.7 The six axes (structural fields) of LOINC codes

Axis	Description	Examples
Component name	Name of the property, analyte, chemical, etc. being measured or observed	Height, pulse, cholesterol, rubella antibodies, lung vital capacity
Property measured	Distinguishes between the different types of quantities that could be measured for a given component/analyte	Mass concentration (mg/dL), substance concentration (mmol/L), arbitrary concentration (IU/mL), mass concentration ratio (protein–creatinine ratio)
Time aspect	Indicates the timing of a measurement or observation point in time or over a period of time	Point sample, 24-h collection, other timed interval
System (or Sample)	The context or system in which the observation was made or the sample type that was used	Patient, fetus, heart, etc.; for lab testing, serum, plasma, cerebrospinal fluid, etc.
Type of scale	The scale of measure being used	Quantitative (typical numeric quantity), ordinal (numbered rank), nominal (identifying number), narrative (free text)
Type of method	Optional description of the methodology used to make the measurement; only included if there is a clinically significant difference between methodologies	Glucose measurement by point-of-care glucometer, as opposed to by serum measurement on the laboratory's blood chemistry analyzer

in 1999. SNOMED-CT is perhaps the most complete clinical terminology available today. It is multi-lingual: currently available in English, Spanish, and Danish, and translations into other languages are in development. It was originally

TABLE 5.8 Examples of LOINC codes used in cytology

Test name	LOINC code	Component	Property	Timing	System	Scale type	Method type
Pap test	10524-7	Microscopic observation	Presence or identify	Point in time	Cervix	Nominal	Cytology stain
ThinPrep Pap test	18500-9	Microscopic observation	Presence or identify	Point in time	Cervix	Nominal	Cytology stain, ThinPrep

developed by the College of American Pathologists (CAP), but is now being developed by the International Health Terminology Standards Development Organization (IHTSDO). It currently contains over 300,000 concepts from most areas of medicine, over 800,000 English language descriptions (including synonyms), and over a million semantic relationships between concepts. SNOMED-CT is based upon a multi-axis system which includes 12 main axes (clinical finding/disorder, procedure/intervention, observable entity, body structure, organism, substance, pharmaceutical/biologic product, specimen, physical object, physical force, event, environment or geographic location, social context, staging, and scales, as well as any special concept). The great power in SNOMED-CT is not so much the entities, but the relationships between entities. For example, it is possible to utilize SNOMED-CT to perform computer-assisted coding in a way that other more limited coding systems cannot enable. However, due to the fact that SNOMED-CT is so flexible, it becomes very complex to encode findings, since there are so many valid choices available. It is recommended that, as with any other computerized coding system, one codes to the highest level of specificity possible.

Chapter 6
Laboratory Information Systems

Ioan C. Cucoranu, Anil V. Parwani, and Liron Pantanowitz

Introduction

The laboratory information system (LIS) is a large, complex system made up of software and hardware that handles electronic data to support laboratory operations. Cytology was one of the first areas of anatomical pathology that embraced informatics, owing to regulations introduced by the Clinical Laboratory Improvement Amendments (CLIA) in 1988. In the cytopathology laboratory, the LIS helps deal with a high volume of specimens, repetitive tasks, and comply with required standards. The LIS provides a mechanism to electronically integrate patient data (e.g., demographics, clinical history, archived pathology reports), facilitate laboratory workflow processes, communicate diagnostic interpretations, assist with billing, capture coding, aid in quality assurance (QA), and connect with other information systems (e.g., hospital information system, electronic medical

I.C. Cucoranu, M.D. (✉) • A.V. Parwani, M.D., Ph.D., M.B.A.
L. Pantanowitz, M.D.
Department of Pathology, University of Pittsburgh Medical Center,
Pittsburgh, PA, USA
e-mail: cucoranuic@upmc.edu; parwaniav@upmc.edu;
pantanowitzl@upmc.edu

L. Pantanowitz and A.V. Parwani (eds.), *Practical Informatics for Cytopathology*, Essentials in Cytopathology 14, DOI 10.1007/978-1-4614-9581-9_6, © Springer Science+Business Media New York 2014

record, billing system). A stand-alone LIS is a system devoted entirely to Anatomical (or Clinical) Pathology (AP-LIS or CP-LIS). Such an LIS is often referred to as a best-of-breed LIS, because of the in depth functionality it offers. While an integrated LIS, one that is used for both Anatomical and Clinical Pathology, may not provide as much functionality the advantage of such an LIS is that the lab has to now only deal with one vendor as well as a single database, log-on, and so forth. Moreover, an integrated LIS eliminates the need to interface data between different laboratory departments. More recently, we have witnessed a larger proportion of labs having to work within enterprise-wide (hospital) information systems (e.g., electronic medical record that includes an LIS module). Finally, there is an Application Service Provider (ASP) model where a lab opts to "rent" an entirely Web-based LIS.

Laboratory Information System Components

The LIS is composed of multiple interrelated hardware components, networking technology and software applications that work together to manage patient related data (Fig. 6.1).

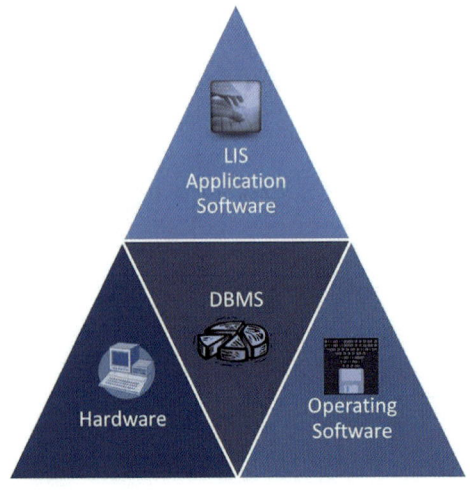

FIG. 6.1 Core components of the LIS (DBMS = database management system)

The hardware and operating system provide the information technology (IT) infrastructure for the LIS. LIS functionality is supported by the database management system (DBMS) and vendor application software.

Hardware

LIS hardware components include computers (servers, work-station personal computers, and terminals), networking equipment and peripheral devices (e.g., printers, fax machines, barcode scanners, digital imaging devices).

Operating Systems

The operating system (OS) is a complex set of programs that manages all the hardware and software resources (program applications). The OS allows the LIS applications to communicate and control the computer hardware resources such as memory, portals, peripheral devices, and networking. The main operating systems currently in use are Microsoft Windows, Mac OS, UNIX, and Linux. A LIS usually provides services to more than one area of the laboratory, supports multiple users with various roles, and includes multiple computers with various configurations. Therefore, multiple operating systems or multiple versions of the same operating system may be in use at any given time. For instance, the main database server computer may have a version of UNIX as its OS while a particular end user's desktop computer may use a version of Microsoft Windows (e.g., Windows 7).

Database Management Systems (DBMS)

Databases are the core of any LIS. They help define standard data definitions and processing procedures. They store all the information related to patients, specimens and test results, as well as information related to various steps in the workflow of the laboratory. These data are stored and organized in files that are structured (typically in a relational database) based on predefined formats and templates. Individual data files are composed of records called data fields or data elements. These electronic databases are managed by specialized software called Database Management System (DBMS), which helps control the access, organization, storage, management, querying and retrieval of data.

Laboratory Information System Application Software

The software layer used to perform predefined laboratory functions is the LIS application software. On the "front end" (user view) laboratory staff interact with this layer of the LIS by using built-in user interfaces. On the "back end" (administrative view) the LIS application software interacts with the DBMS or with computer/network hardware, to communicate the user's commands.

Laboratory Information System Architecture

Multiple computers and devices (e.g., lab instruments, fax machines) are interconnected by networks that permit the transmission of electronic information and data exchange between LIS computers, or between the LIS and other computer systems. There are two main types of architecture used for this purpose: mainframe and client–server models.

Mainframe Architecture

This type of LIS architecture has a central computer, called a mainframe, which is in charge of all LIS functions and transactions. The mainframe computer hosts the LIS database and application software. Users access the LIS by using "dumb" terminals. These are computers with no internal

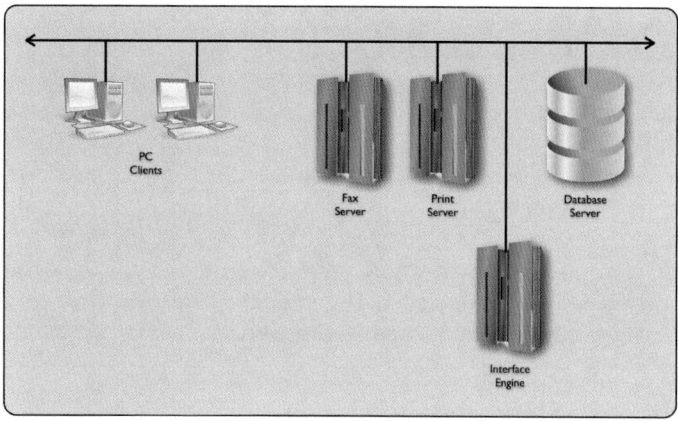

Fɪɢ. 6.2 Client–server LIS architecture

microprocessor. Hence, they do not have data processing capabilities. Their function is to merely display data and allow users to interact with the mainframe through a keyboard. They are connected to the mainframe via intermediate computers called terminal servers. While this type of architecture is relatively simple, it has limited flexibility and is therefore infrequently used today.

Client–Server Architecture

This type of LIS architecture is more commonly used by laboratories today. With this type of network, applications that perform tasks are distributed between servers (computer hosts that provide a resource or service) and clients (computers that request a service, but do not share their resources) (Fig. 6.2). Examples of resources include data, computer processing, printers, and storage. The servers communicate with middle-tier software (the back end) to retrieve and store information from a database. Although there is decentralized organization and increased complexity, users prefer to work with such peripheral computers (clients) as they have a more friendly user interface. This type of set up does require greater maintenance, as software and updates need to be installed on each peripheral computer. To improve this demand for ongoing maintenance, some laboratories employ "thin client" architecture. With thin clients (network computers) the bulk of the data processing occurs on the server. In contrast, a thick (or fat) client is one that performs the bulk of the processing on the peripheral computer. Thin client set-up simplifies administration and make it easier to distribute software updates, because client computers are now controlled and standardized more centrally.

Core Laboratory Information System Elements

A few components such as dictionaries, worksheets, and interfaces are indispensable for LIS functions related to laboratory workflow and data management.

Dictionaries

Dictionaries are tables (also called maintenance files). They are components of the LIS database that play a significant role in defining data formats, structures, and rules. Various types of data definitions are predefined in dictionaries. Examples of dictionaries include tables that contain specimen part types, list of doctor's names, a menu of special stains, diagnoses used for reporting (e.g., The Bethesda System terminology), billing codes, users passwords, and so on. Dictionaries can constrain the entry of data in certain fields to discrete, predefined values. This provides standardization. They can also be used to define rules or calculations that need to be applied to data. Dictionaries may be prebuilt by the vendor, but typically the lab defines and maintains entries to meet specific needs.

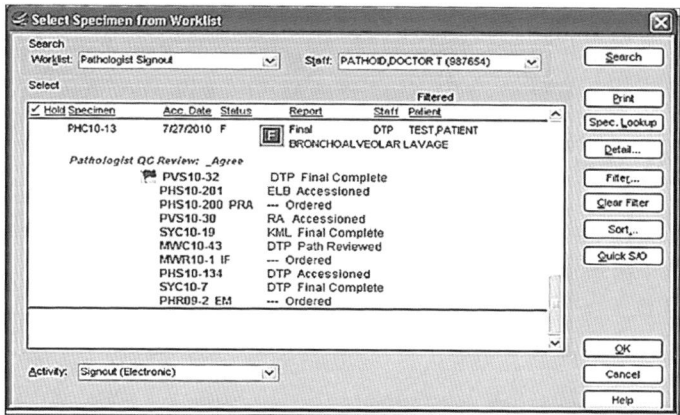

FIG. 6.3 Screenshot from a test LIS system showing an example of a pathologist's signout worklist of a BAL case. This case shares several other specimens being handled in the lab (some being ordered, others accessioned, or complete and finalized)

Worklists

LIS worklists can have flexible formats and are used for many functions, such as keeping an active list of cases assigned to a pathologist that they have to sign-out (Fig. 6.3). These worklists define specimen workflow in the cytopathology laboratory, and are also known as work logs (e.g., list of cases to be stained, to add on HPV testing).

Interfaces

Interfaces are software and hardware components that allow the LIS to connect with other information systems (e.g., billing system) or lab instruments (e.g., Pap test imager) (Fig. 6.4). Interface engines translate electronic messages (e.g., orders, results) that are being transmitted and thereby facilitate automated communication. When selecting and purchasing a new LIS it is important to evaluate the system's interface

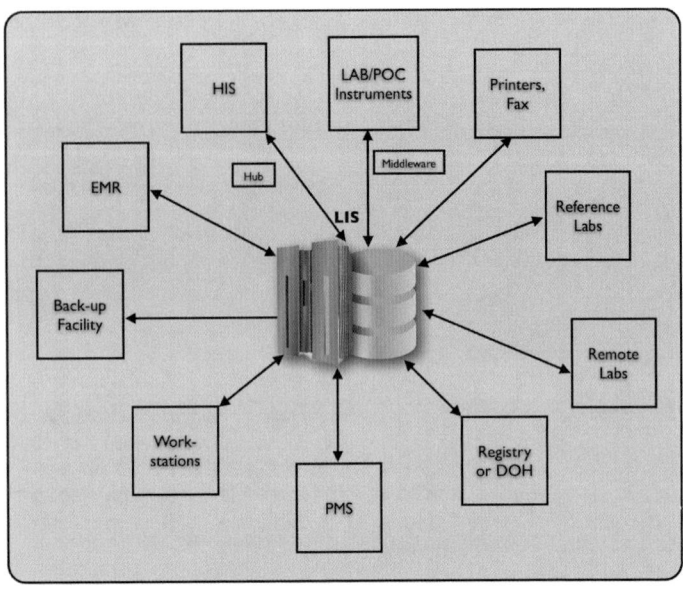

FIG. 6.4 Schematic showing laboratory information system (LIS) connectivity with several devices and other information systems. *DOH* = department of health, *EMR* = electronic medical record, *HIS* = hospital information system, *LAB* = laboratory, *PMS* = practice management system, *POC* = point-of-care

capability. The Health Level 7 (HL7) standard is the main communication protocol used to transmit electronic information between information systems in the health care setting.

Laboratory Information System Functions

The LIS performs several critical functions (Table 6.1). When dealing with large specimen volumes, especially Pap tests, it has become especially critical to standardize operations and rely on computers. Perhaps one of the most important tasks for the LIS is workflow management in the cytology lab (Fig. 6.5). The LIS has allowed labs to take advantage of automation. For example, in the pre-analytical phase, patient

TABLE 6.1 Laboratory information system functions

- Workflow management
- Specimen tracking
- Data entry
- Reporting
- Archiving data
- Assistance with regulatory compliance
- Code capture
- Interfacing with other systems
- Billing information
- QA measures

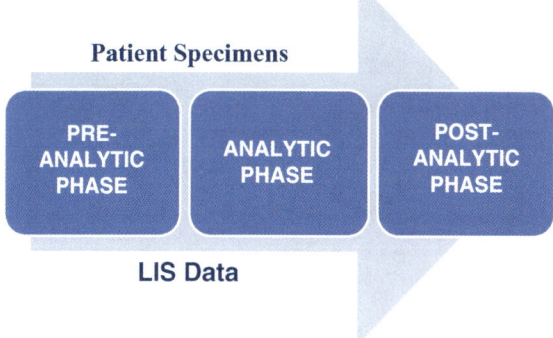

Patient Specimens

| PRE-ANALYTIC PHASE | ANALYTIC PHASE | POST-ANALYTIC PHASE |

LIS Data

FIG. 6.5 LIS functions and laboratory workflow. Data in the LIS gets managed in alliance with the processing of patient specimens, their derivatives (blocks, slides) and reporting. This includes the pre-analytic (e.g., specimen accession), analytic (e.g., interpretation, ancillary testing, results entry), and post-analytic (e.g., reporting, corrected results) phases of the test process

demographics can be automatically fed into the LIS from the Hospital Information System (HIS) by means of an Admission, Discharge, Transfer (ADT) interface. The LIS also makes data entry, reporting, and archiving of information much

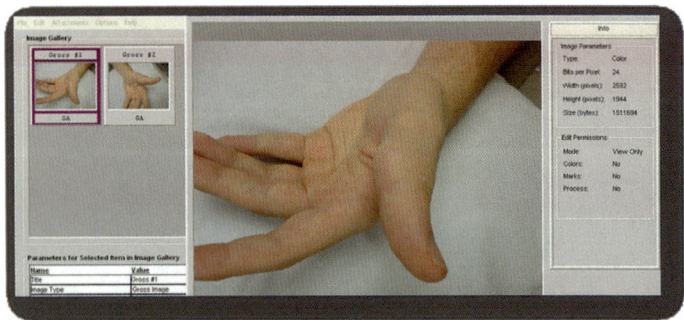

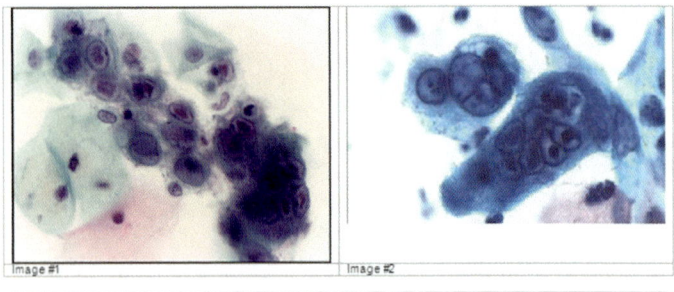

FIG. 6.6 LIS image management. The *top image* shows an example of an integrated digital photo acquired in a FNA clinic that is stored within the LIS image gallery. The *bottom image* is an example of a cytology report with embedded images

easier to perform than traditional paper-based systems. Code capture and billing in the LIS has improved compliance and allows for quicker reimbursement. In cytopathology, leveraging the LIS electronic database helps with regulatory compliance, as well as with quality assurance (QA) and quality control (QC) to detect, correct, and reduce errors. Newer functionality being integrated into the LIS includes voice

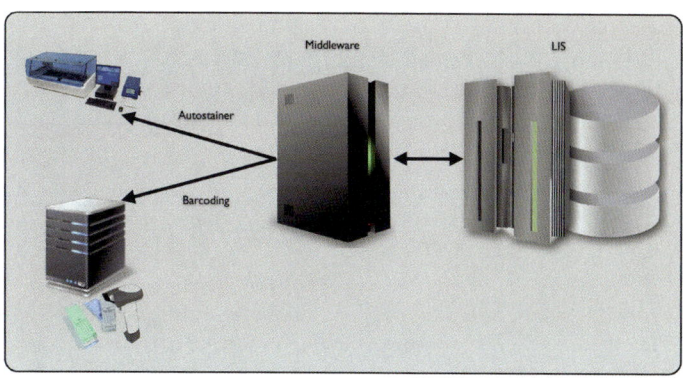

Fɪɢ. 6.7 Diagram showing middleware as computer equipment located between the LIS and laboratory instruments or devices

recognition, synoptic reporting (mainly for surgical pathology), and digital imaging (Fig. 6.6). As a result of the increasing number of institutions and physician practices now utilizing an electronic medical record (EMR), and looking to achieve "meaningful use" (refer to Chap. 13) with their certified EMRs, there is greater demand for LIS-EMR connectivity. This has also resulted in greater competition for informatics resources (financial and IT staff). Moreover, informatics staff will accordingly need to participate in creating EMR decision support tools (e.g., drug-lab result alerts), as well as maintenance of electronic transmission issues (e.g., failed orders, downtime) and problems related to the display of electronic pathology reports (e.g., format) in these downstream systems.

Middleware

Middleware is hardware and/or software inserted between lab instruments and the LIS (Fig. 6.7). Middleware not only connects legacy to newer systems but also allows data exchange/management that the LIS cannot handle. Therefore, it is a cost-effective way to add functionality to a legacy LIS. Middleware can be added at the instrument level (e.g., on-board instrument data management software) or LIS level. This approach has demonstrated success at facilitating lab automation, improving productivity (e.g., reduced staff needs), speeding up workflow, and promoting standardization with fewer errors.

Laboratory Information System Selection

Cytology does not usually have a stand-alone LIS. Rather, cytology is typically managed using a highly customized module of the AP-LIS. Therefore, when selecting a LIS the needs of the cytology lab are typically added to those of the entire pathology laboratory. Ideally, cytology leadership should be involved in the decision-making and selection process for a new LIS. This process typically involves the following steps:

1. Creation of a project team with a designated leader
2. Assessment of needs and requirements (e.g., gap analysis, ranking desired features)
3. Viable candidate identification (screening LIS vendor qualifications)
4. Requesting vendor system and corporate information using documents (Table 6.2)
5. Cost quotations (request for price quotation)
6. Telephone reference checks, onsite demonstrations, and site visits to existing users
7. Contract negotiations

TABLE 6.2 Documents used to obtain vendor information

RFI (request for information)	Request addressed to a potential vendor to inquire about products and services available.
RFP (request for proposal)	Invitation for vendors to submit a detailed proposal on their product/service in response to specific stated requirements.
RPQ (request for price quotation)	Document used to solicit vendor price quotations based on major requirements and operational statistics.

Laboratory Information System Implementation

System implementation (or deployment) refers to the installation and testing of an information system. This covers a broad spectrum of activities ranging from planning, full system testing, possible workflow modification (and even new procedures), formal go-live of the new system, resolution of application issues during and after the implementation period, and documentation. Validation is the documented process of assuring that the LIS performs exactly what it is designed to do in a consistent and reproducible manner. Critical tasks include adequate testing of interfaces, data conversion, pre-live validation, and final system acceptance. The success of LIS implementation relies heavily on project planning, effective management, users (lab staff) involvement, resource allocation, focused execution, and end-users training. When one or more of these factors is deficient, project delays, cost overruns as well as staff and administration frustration could be encountered. A common cause for implementation delay is when staff with other full time job responsibilities are assigned to the LIS implementation team. Therefore, realistic personnel assignments should be made. The vendor of the system usually plays a prominent role. An implementation plan provided by the vendor can be used as a template and modified to accommodate the laboratory environment. When in-house staff have insufficient experience regarding LIS implementation (and even selection), consultation services should be considered.

Chapter 7
Laboratory Information System Operations and Regulations

Ioan C. Cucoranu, Anil V. Parwani, and Liron Pantanowitz

Introduction

The mission of the computerized laboratory information system (LIS) is to manage laboratory workflow, patient information, and deliver results for patient clinical management accurately and in a timely manner. In recent years, laboratories has been under pressure to enhance their workflow (e.g., Lean initiatives, automation, and tracking) and to expand the menu of tests offered, to remain competitive, while at the same time improving their quality of service. In order to accomplish this, the LIS needs to remain continuously operational with minimal or no downtime. Moreover, LIS staff needs to ensure that all operations are compliant with mandated rules and regulations. Optimal LIS operations depend on having adequate, dedicated and skilled informatics staff.

I.C. Cucoranu, M.D. (✉) • A.V. Parwani, M.D., Ph.D., M.B.A.
L. Pantanowitz, M.D.
Department of Pathology, University of Pittsburgh Medical Center, Pittsburgh, PA, USA
e-mail: cucoranuic@upmc.edu; parwaniav@upmc.edu; pantanowitzl@upmc.edu

L. Pantanowitz and A.V. Parwani (eds.), *Practical Informatics for Cytopathology*, Essentials in Cytopathology 14, DOI 10.1007/978-1-4614-9581-9_7,
© Springer Science+Business Media New York 2014

TABLE 7.1 LIS team operations

• Help desk support
• Change control
• System security
• System data backup
• Interface monitoring
• Manage unscheduled and scheduled downtimes
• Database maintenance
• Software upgrades
• Administrative and management reporting
• Budgeting and cost analyses
• System validation
• External information services department initiatives
• Documentation
• Evaluate new products
• Participate in quality improvement programs
• Partake in new internal and external projects

Such individuals can have a laboratory background (e.g., laboratory technologist or manager) or come from information technology (IT) services (e.g., information analysts, programmers, network engineers). Communication and cooperation between LIS staff and IT personnel is critical for successful maintenance of the LIS. Table 7.1 lists some of the key operations the LIS team handles.

Help Desk Support

Personnel involved with supporting information systems and related technology may have different roles and responsibilities at different institutions. LIS help desk support specialists provide technical assistance with personal computers (workstations), operating systems, LIS-related applications (e.g., password help), and sometimes with peripheral devices (e.g., digital cameras) or software (e.g., voice recognition software) used in the laboratory. They may also be asked to train users on the proper use of these components. Help desk support software applications are available to manage large volumes of requests. Support processes and procedures that are planned, well managed, and friendly can minimize customer frustration.

Change Control

Change control is a process that ensures that changes are recorded, evaluated, authorized, and monitored in a controlled and coordinated fashion. This applies to any changes (revisions, alterations, additions, enhancements, or upgrades) performed on hardware or software. These changes may be required by the vendor, IT services or by the laboratory. Documentation of all changes is mandated by regulatory bodies such as the College of American Pathologists (CAP). LIS managers are responsible for change control documentation. Commercial software for change control process management is available. A list of items required to be documented is presented in Table 7.2. Good planning upfront, handy policies and standard operation procedures (SOPs), as well as adherence to change control processes can potentially prevent the laboratory from making costly mistakes such as system crashes, project failures, security breaches and data corruption.

Laboratory Information System Security

The LIS must provide users with rapid access to complete and accurate patient results while safeguarding patient privacy and confidentiality. It is important to ensure that this information is available and can be accessed only by authorized personnel. The LIS administrator is responsible

TABLE 7.2 Change control documentation

Documentation items	Explanation of change
Description of change	Detailed explanation of the change performed
Reason for change	Need and benefits for the performed change
Persons responsible for change implementation	Allows for identification of the personnel that actually performed the change
Change category	Hardware, software, process or procedural
Degree of change	Minor versus major—based on overall impact on the LIS, health care IT system and laboratory, including cost
Change sign-off	Identifies the person responsible for the overall change
Risk assessment	Allows for problems that may incur as result of the change to be assessed, and planning for resolution if such problems occur
Evaluation and monitoring of the implemented changes	Evaluates outcome and determines the success of change implementation

for system security, which includes user access, privileges, auditing and enforcement of certain regulations (e.g., HIPAA). The security level and access to the LIS is based on the functions a user needs in order to perform their laboratory assigned tasks. HIPAA security rules (see later) mandate that covered entities determine risks due to threats and implement adequate measures to protect patient information. User access (login) relies on user identification (ID) and a password. Password strength is a function of length, complexity, and unpredictability. Biometrics is also beginning to be used in the health care setting. These are unique and measurable characteristics of a human being that allow automatic recognition or identity verification (e.g., fingerprints, retina pattern recognition, speech scans, and even sometimes DNA). Information system security requires risk analysis to assess

LIS vulnerability and planning for loss of information stored in databases. Intrusion detection and audit software may be used for this process. Risk assessment is mandated by HIPAA and is usually the responsibility of an appointed security officer. The LIS manager should be familiar with the various types of potential threats and is responsible for training users to prevent security breaches. Computer viruses and other malicious computer programs (e.g., malware, spyware) should be prevented at all costs. This can be achieved in part by using anti-malware (antivirus) software.

System Backup

Disaster recovery is a set of processes, policies and procedures that can enable recovery and continuation of critical IT infrastructure after a disaster. Disasters may be natural (e.g., floods, fire) or human-induced (e.g., power failure, hacker, hazardous chemical spill, bioterrorism). A disaster recovery plan is also referred to as a "business continuity plan." Precautionary measures include regularly scheduled data backup, replication of data to off-site locations, use of redundant storage technology such as redundant array of independent disks (RAID), uninterruptible power supplies (UPS), and backup power generation. Backup of LIS data should include patient data (e.g., automatically scheduled during off-peak hours on a daily basis), LIS database master tables (e.g., at least monthly), and operating systems.

Management Reporting

A modern LIS is capable of generating automated or on-demand management reports such as documentation for regulatory compliance, quality assurance, or for monitoring performance and productivity (e.g., turn-around time, abnormal results, reimbursement). Chapter 9 provides an overview of such reporting that is used to support the quality management program of a cytology lab.

Regulations

There are a number of regulatory and accreditation agencies that may evaluate the LIS during a mandatory laboratory inspection. In the United States, these include the Center for Medicaid Services (CMS), Office of Civil Rights (OCR) for HIPAA, The Joint Commission (TJC), College of American Pathologists (CAP), and Commission on Office Laboratory Accreditation (COLA) for CLIA'88. ISO 15189 is an internationally recognized laboratory accreditation standard, developed by the International Organization for Standardization, which specifies the quality management system and competency requirements unique to medical laboratories. Software solutions (e.g., electronic document control) can help medical laboratories achieve ISO 15189 certification.

Health Insurance Portability and Accountability Act (HIPAA)

HIPAA was signed by President Bill Clinton in 1996. The act includes several titles (Fig. 7.1). Title II (also known as the Administrative Simplification provisions) is most germane to laboratorians including cytologists because it deals with the exchange of electronic data, privacy, and security in health care. The intent of these standards is to improve (the efficiency and effectiveness of) the US health care system by encouraging the widespread use of electronic data interchange (EDI). It also helps control fraud and abuse. HIPAA (1) defines several policies, procedures, and guidelines for maintaining the privacy and security of individually identifiable health information and (2) outlines the offenses and penalties that may be incurred for violations. These rules apply to "covered entities" (e.g., health care providers, plans, and clearinghouses). As per the requirements of Title II, the

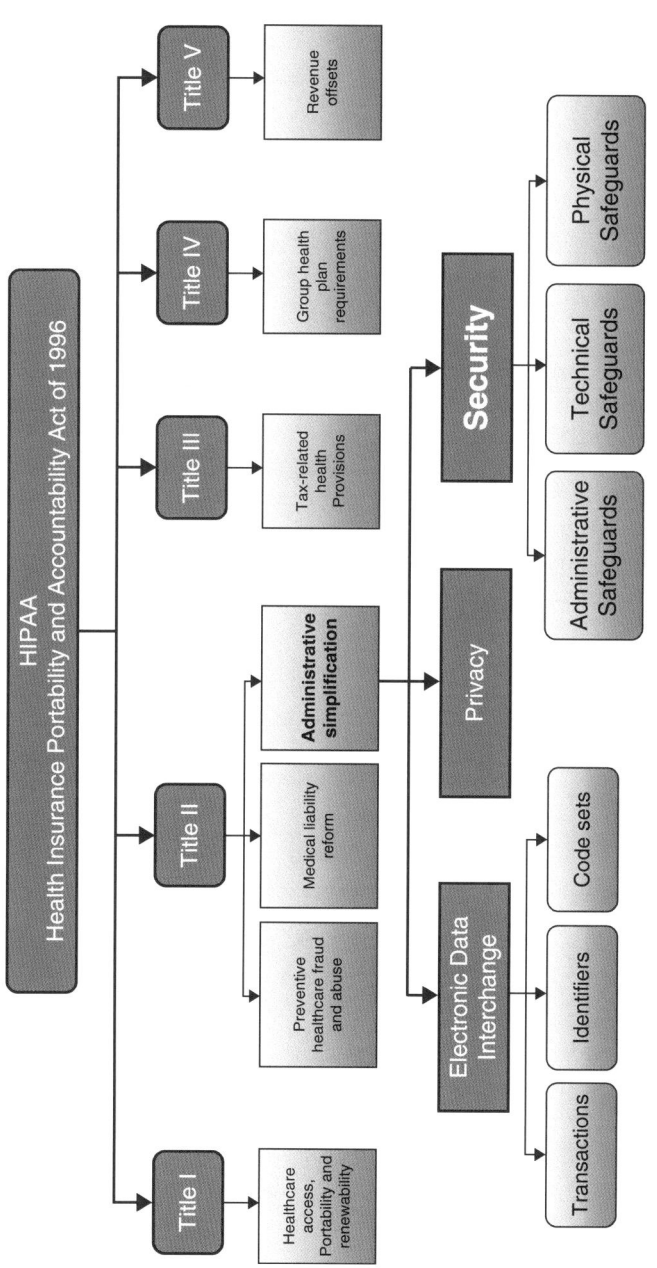

Fig. 7.1 Overview of HIPAA

Department of Health and Human Services (HHS) has promulgated the following five rules:

- *Transactions and Code Sets Rule*. This rule states that HIPAA-covered entities are required to use standardized HIPAA electronic transactions.
- *Privacy Rule*. This rule regulates the use and disclosure of Protected Health Information (PHI) held by covered entities. A covered entity may disclose PHI to facilitate treatment, payment, or health care operations without a patient's express written authorization. However, for all other disclosures of PHI, a written authorization from the individual must be obtained. Covered entities need to also notify individuals of how their PHI is used.
- *Security Rule*. This rule deals specifically with electronic PHI (ePHI). It specifies three types of security safeguards required for compliance: administrative, physical, and technical (see below). For each safeguard there are required and addressable (more flexible) implementation specifications.
- *Unique Identifiers Rule*. This rule required HIPAA covered entities to use a National Provider Identifier (NPI) to identify covered health care providers in electronic communications.
- *Enforcement Rule*. This rule determines civil money penalties for violating HIPAA rules and establishes procedures for investigations and hearings for HIPAA violations. Commonly reported violations include misuse of PHI, failure to have protection in place for ePHI, patients' inability to access their health information, and using or disclosing more than the minimum necessary PHI.

Administrative Safeguards

Health Insurance Portability and Accountability Act (HIPAA)

The HIPAA Security Rule mandates the following nine administrative safeguards to protect ePHI:

- Security management functions that require implementation of risk analysis, risk management, sanction policies, and information system activity reviews.
- Assigned security responsibility to an official.
- Workforce security with addressable functions for work authorization and supervision, workforce clearance procedures, and termination procedures.
- Information access management standards to address access authorization.
- Security awareness and training standards that require periodic security reminders, protection from malicious software, log-in monitoring, and password management.
- Security incident procedures.
- Contingency plans to cover data backup, disaster recovery, and emergency mode operation.
- Periodic technical and non-technical evaluations.
- Business associated contracts.

Physical Safeguards

Health Insurance Portability and Accountability Act (HIPAA)

Physical safeguards control physical access to protect against inappropriate access to protected data. The following four required standards help protect the LIS, related equipment, and buildings from unauthorized intrusions or from natural and environmental hazards:

- Facility access control with addressable functions including contingency operations, facility security plan, access control and validation, or maintenance records.
- Workstation use and required policies.
- Workstation security based on restriction of access only to authorized users.
- Devices and media control based on disposal, media reuse, accountability, data backup, and storage.

Technical Safeguards

Health Insurance Portability and Accountability Act (HIPAA)

These safeguards are designed to control access to computer systems and enable covered entities to protect communications containing PHI transmitted electronically over open networks from being intercepted by anyone other than the intended recipient. Required automated processes that are used for data protection and data access control include:

- Access based on unique user identification, emergency access procedures, automatic log-off, data encryption and decryption.
- Audit control to examine system utilization and access.
- Data integrity based on authentication of ePHI.
- Persons or entities authentication.
- Security of data transmission based on integrity control and encryption.

Chapter 8
Reporting

Liron Pantanowitz

Introduction

The cytology report represents the clinical product of the laboratory. The intent is to accurately communicate a diagnosis to healthcare providers in order to support appropriate and timely patient management. Newer information technology (IT) has allowed laboratories to become more paperless, exploit instrument interfaces, and transmit reports to the electronic medical record (EMR) as well as the Internet (e.g., patient portals). One of the main functions of a laboratory information system (LIS) is to facilitate electronic reporting and transmission of lab reports. Cytology reports contain largely textual narrative information, unlike Clinical Pathology reports (e.g., chemistry) where mostly quantitative data is reported. Therefore, it is important that the information in cytology reports is presented in a concise and easy-to-read format that will also not hamper their electronic transmission and downstream display.

L. Pantanowitz, M.D. (✉)
Department of Pathology, University of Pittsburgh Medical Center,
Pittsburgh, PA, USA
e-mail: pantanowitzl@upmc.edu

L. Pantanowitz and A.V. Parwani (eds.), *Practical Informatics*
for Cytopathology, Essentials in Cytopathology 14,
DOI 10.1007/978-1-4614-9581-9_8,
© Springer Science+Business Media New York 2014

Report Elements

Both the content and format of the cytology report are important. A typical LIS-generated report consists of a header
(patient, submitting physician, laboratory, and specimen
details), diagnosis field (interpretation), and footer (optional
notes or comments). Some laboratories may opt to tailor their
reports for aesthetic and marketing purposes. According to
the Clinical Laboratory Improvement Amendments (CLIA)
standards in the USA, cytology reports (paper and/or electronic) are required to include the following data elements:

- Patient name and unique identifying number
- Patient age and/or date of birth
- Date of collection
- Accession number
- Name of physician and/or clinic
- Name of responsible reviewing pathologist
- Name and address of the performing laboratory
- Report date
- Test performed
- Specimen anatomic source and/or type

If a laboratory fails to display these required elements in
their cytology reports, it may result in citations. Hence, when
electronic interfaces are being established, it is important to
verify that cytology reports displayed in the EMR contain all
of these elements.

Standardized Reporting

In Cytopathology, The Bethesda System for Pap tests and
thyroid fine needle aspirations (FNA) has helped provide
some degree of standardization for reporting. The British
Society for Clinical Cytology (BSCC) also has a reporting
system for Pap tests that is aligned with The Bethesda System.
Table 8.1 summarizes the advantages of such standardized
reporting. Drop-down menus (tables) in the LIS can be built

TABLE 8.1 Advantages of standardized reporting

Conducive to rapid electronic sign out
Improves communication among cytologists, surgical pathologists and healthcare providers
Promotes clear management guidelines
Facilitates data extraction, exchange and analysis
Inspires multi-institutional studies
Offers a mechanism for modification and reform
Improves patient care

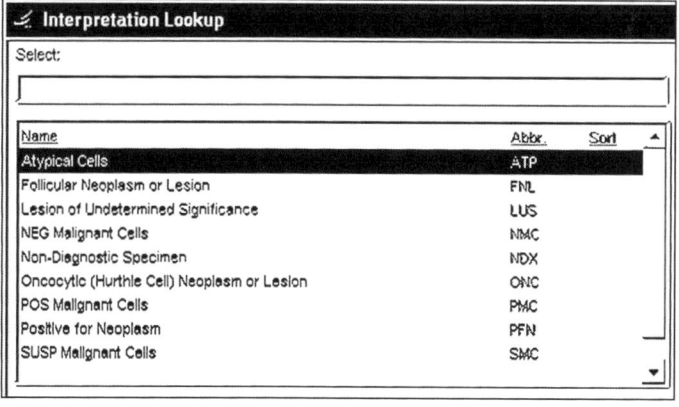

FIG. 8.1 Screenshot of a LIS drop-down list for reporting thyroid FNA cases

to restrict user interpretations to those recommended in The Bethesda System (Fig. 8.1).

Electronic Reporting

Electronic reporting needs to be efficient, safe, and convenient. Reporting should accommodate the workflow in the cytology lab. Therefore, after a cytotechnologist has screened

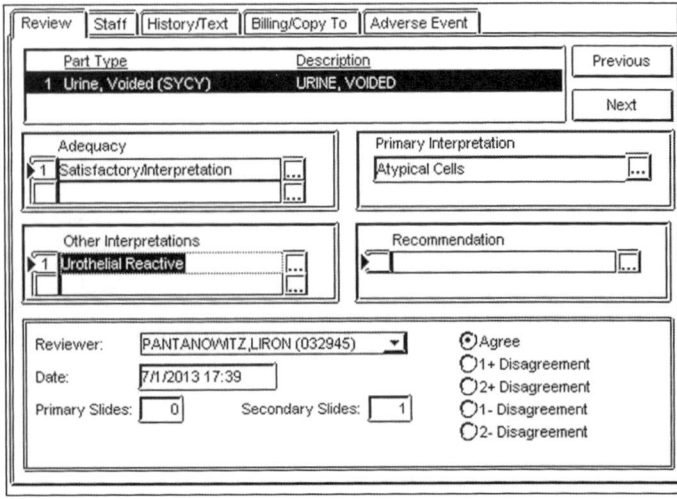

FIG. 8.2 Screenshot showing the required fields in a LIS to enter specimen adequacy, interpretation, number of slides reviewed and agreement/disagreement between cytopathologist and cytotechnologist

a case assigned to them, they will need to enter their final diagnosis into the LIS and then either (1) electronically sign this case out if it was a negative Pap test, or (2) refer the case (e.g., abnormal Pap test or non-gynecological specimen) to a pathologist's worklist for their subsequent final review and electronic sign out. By using an electronic signature (e-signature) in the LIS a cytology user indicates that they legally adopt the contents of the electronic report being signed out. Before a cytology report can be signed out, several key data points (fields) will need to be completed including specimen adequacy, primary interpretation, number of slides reviewed, and sometimes the agreement/level of disagreement between cytopathologist and cytotechnologist (Fig. 8.2). Along with limiting the choices available in drop down lists, this required data entry feature helps improve the entry of valid data into the LIS. To avoid causing interface errors, erratic displays, or printing problems when transmitting electronic reports as a Health Level 7 (HL7) message, it is best to avoid the following characters: vertical bar or pipe (|), caret (^), ampersand (&), at (@), and tilde (~).

Chapter 9
Quality Management

Liron Pantanowitz, Luke T. Wiehagen, and R. Marshall Austin

Introduction

An ongoing quality management program designed to monitor and evaluate the overall quality of the laboratory testing process helps detect, reduce, and correct deficiencies. Quality control (QC) procedures help ensure that the preparation, interpretation, and reporting of cytology specimens meets specified quality criteria. Quality assurance (QA) is a retrospective tool that measures the success of specific processes. In the USA, the Clinical Laboratory Improvement Amendments of 1988 (CLIA '88) are federally mandated standards that serve as the foundation of cytology QC/QA. To obtain a CLIA certificate a laboratory must be accredited (and inspected) by The Joint Commission (TJC), formerly called the Joint Commission of Healthcare Organizations

L. Pantanowitz, M.D. (✉) • L.T. Wiehagen, B.S.
Department of Pathology, University of Pittsburgh Medical Center, Pittsburgh, PA, USA
e-mail: pantanowtizl@upmc.edu

R.M. Austin, M.D., Ph.D.
Department of Pathology, Magee-Womens Hospital, University of Pittsburgh Medical Center, Pittsburgh, PA, USA

L. Pantanowitz and A.V. Parwani (eds.), *Practical Informatics for Cytopathology*, Essentials in Cytopathology 14, DOI 10.1007/978-1-4614-9581-9_9,
© Springer Science+Business Media New York 2014

TABLE 9.1 Benefits of electronic data

- Standardized reporting
- Rapid transmission of information
- Integration of multiple records
- Easy and efficient data analysis
- Timely financial transactions
- Decreased storage space requirements
- Multiple user access to stored information

(JCAHO), or the College of American Pathologists (CAP). To perform QA activities laboratories need access to electronic data, typically obtained from the laboratory information system (LIS), and computer tools to analyze these data (Table 9.1). Sometimes this may involve extracting LIS data into external software applications (e.g., spreadsheets). A cytology lab, for example, needs to maintain records of their annual number of cases, specimen types processed, and volume of cases stratified by interpretation. They also need to monitor several screening and performance indicators (e.g., cytologic–histologic correlation, workload limits). The LIS is often utilized to monitor the overall test process which includes pre-analytic (e.g., test requisitions, cytopreparation), analytic (e.g., screening and diagnostic performance), and post-analytic (e.g., test reports) phases. It is also important for the lab to maintain records of their quality management surveillance. Clearly, in order to meet current quality management demands, cytologists today need to be computer-savvy and educated about informatics.

Quality Indicators

Quality indicators of diagnostic accuracy for Pap tests include rescreening measures. Rescreening is mandated by CLIA in the USA. This includes prospective and retrospective rescreening of selected cases. QC rescreening is most useful for detecting screening errors, as opposed to diagnostic errors. Some international studies have shown that rapid rescreening or prescreening of 100 % of cases may be more effective at detecting false negative Pap test results than 10 % random rescreening or rescreening on the basis of clinical (high-risk) criteria (Tavares et al. 2008). However, this may not be practical in a large cytology laboratory involved in screening a high volume of cases or one with limited staff. Other potential quality indicators (monitors) a cytology laboratory can chose to evaluate include rejected and unsatisfactory specimens, cytopreparation problems, turnaround time, and client satisfaction (Clary et al. 2013).

Prospective Rescreen

This requirement in the USA involves a prospective 10 % rescreen (reexamination prior to reporting) of each cytotechnologist's (not pathologist) Pap test cases selected both randomly and including high-risk women based on criteria established by the Medical Director. The LIS can be leveraged to mark cases for QC on a lab-wide basis. The LIS needs to be configured so that a case selected for QC cannot be reported out until the rescreen is complete. If a cytotechnologist is new they may require a higher rescreening ratio. The LIS can be instrumental in adjusting these individual thresholds. The LIS can also be used to generate reports to verify that each cytotechnologist has met this minimum requirement of 10 % QC rescreen for their negative Pap test cases.

Retrospective Rescreen

CLIA regulations in the USA mandate a retrospective review of all negative Pap tests for the last 5 years (so-called "5-year look back") for which current Pap tests are diagnosed with a high grade squamous intraepithelial lesion (HSIL) or above (i.e., cancer). These archival cases are searchable using the LIS. These cases provide educational feedback for cytotechnologists and pathologists. Although the CLIA look back requirement is triggered by abnormal cytology results, in our experience more educationally valuable material may be discovered when the "5-year look back" requirement is extended to include histopathologic diagnoses of cervical intraepithelial neoplasia (CIN) 2 and 3, adenocarcinoma in situ (AIS), and cervical cancer reported in the LIS (Austin and Zhao 2011).

Pre-sign-out Quality Assurance Tool (PQAT)

For some laboratory information systems (e.g., CoPathPlus, Cerner) a PQAT tool automatically and randomly selects an adjustable percentage (e.g., 10 %) of non-gynecological cytopathology cases for review before release (sign-out) of the final report by pathologists. Selected cases get assigned to a second QA cytopathologist for review. The PQAT provides a prospective, LIS-driven, peer review mechanism to prevent diagnostic errors from occurring and corrective action to be taken prior to reporting. Agreement and disagreements with this tool can be tracked in the LIS (Fig. 9.1).

Cytologic–Histologic Correlation (CHC)

For QC purposes, cytology laboratories need to compare their cytologic diagnoses with available subsequent histopathologic findings. This needs to be conducted for both gynecologic (Pap test and cervical biopsy reports) (Table 9.2) and non-gynecologic cases. CHC is believed to be a monitor of the overall "system." Unfortunately, there is no standard method to collect this data, nor are there metrics for interlaboratory comparison. CHC can be performed in real time and/or retrospectively (e.g., 3 or 6 monthly). If significant disparities exist, these need to be resolved. In our experience with gynecologic cytology, correlation reviews are most productively performed in "real time" when signing out histopathologic specimens with earlier cytology results.

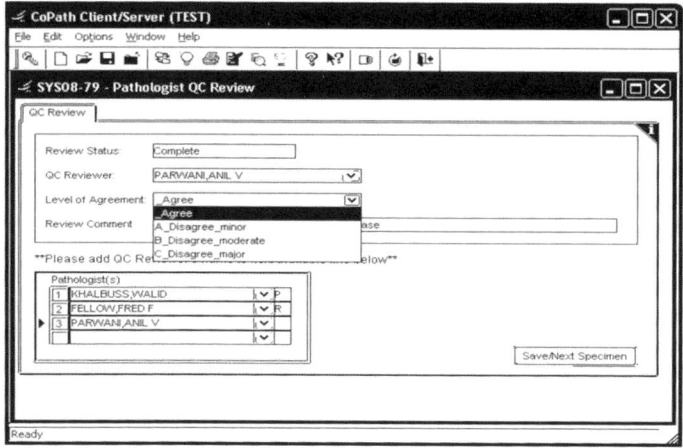

Fig. 9.1 LIS screenshot showing agreement between the QC reviewer and primary pathologist (image courtesy of Anil Parwani, Pittsburgh, PA, USA)

Assessments can focus both on whether or not the histopathologic findings reflect the earlier cytologic findings, as well as on whether or not the cytologic findings warrant additional diagnostic procedures. In our opinion, the most important retrospective quality improvement reviews are on non-correlation cases where either a cytology or histopathologic result of high grade dysplasia (CIN2/3/AIS) or cervical cancer are paired with a non-correlating result of negative or CIN1 (Zhao et al. 2009).

Pap Test Ratios

Apart from monitoring the rates for frequencies of diagnostic categories (e.g., atypical cells of undetermined significance or ASCUS), for Pap tests a cytology lab may monitor specific ratios including the ASCUS/SIL (SIL = squamous intraepithelial lesion) ratio (Renshaw et al. 2009) and ASCUS/HPV DNA positivity rates (Table 9.3) (Tworek et al. 2007; Cibas et al. 2008) (Fig. 9.2). It is extremely important for data on

TABLE 9.2 Typical cytologic–histologic correlation contingency table used for evaluating Pap tests

Time period	Cytologic diagnosis (Pap tests)	Histologic diagnosis (Cervix histopathology)					
		Negative	Atypical	LSIL	HSIL	Carcinoma	Total
Quarter (1–4)	NILM						
	ASC-US						
	ASC-H						
	AGC						
	LSIL						
	HSIL						
	Cancer						

TABLE 9.3 Possible reasons for various ASCUS/SIL and ASCUS/HPV rates (modified from Cibas et al. 2008)

ASCUS/SIL	ASCUS/HPV	Possible explanation
Increased	Normal	Interpreting reactive or SIL cases as ASCUS
Increased	Increased	Interpreting SIL cases as ASCUS
Increased	Decreased	Interpreting reactive cases as ASCUS
Normal	Decreased	Interpreting reactive cases as ASCUS or ASCUS as SIL
Normal	Increased	Interpreting ASCUS as reactive or SIL as ASCUS
Decreased	Normal	Interpreting ASCUS either as reactive and/or SIL
Decreased	Increased	Interpreting SIL as ASCUS and ASCUS as reactive
Decreased	Decreased	Interpreting reactive cases as ASCUS or ASCUS as SIL

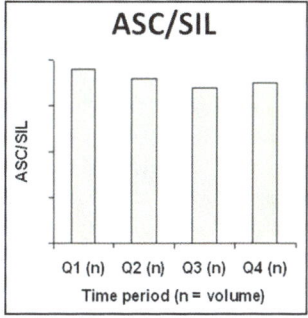 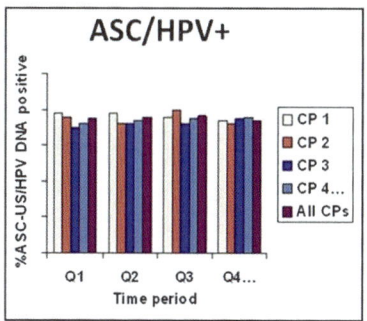

Fɪɢ. 9.2 Graphic representation of (*left*) ASC/SIL ratios for four time quarters (Q1 to Q4) and (*right*) ASC/HPV rates for individual cytopathologists (CP) for four quarters (image courtesy of Dr. Robert Goulart, Springfield, MA, USA)

HPV-positive ASCUS rates to be age-stratified, as HPV rates decrease significantly after age 30 years (Tworek et al. 2007). Some have argued that ASCUS/SIL ratios may serve as better benchmarks than individual diagnostic rates; however, limited data are available linking reported national CAP benchmark ratios to important quality outcomes such as screening sensitivity for detection of high grade precancers and cancers. For example, even if a high ASCUS rate is due to screening a high-risk population, it has been argued that the ASCUS/SIL of the lab should still fall within the national median level (Cibas et al. 2008). Interestingly, data from Canada linking ASCUS/SIL ratios to screening sensitivity (calculated by 100 % rescreening) has indicated that ASCUS/SIL ratios of less than 1.5 may be a surrogate marker of inadequate screening sensitivity (Renshaw et al. 2009). Unfortunately, CAP benchmark data place nearly half of US laboratories in this group (Eversole et al. 2010). Furthermore, screening sensitivity exceeding 95 % was documented in the Canadian study only with outlier ASC/SIL ratios over 3.0 (Eversole et al. 2010). Such ratios may offer a useful QC monitor, but need to be much more clearly linked to important quality outcomes. In our opinion, attention should also be focused on monitoring HPV test performance associated with clinically significant histopathologic outcomes such as CIN2, CIN3, AIS, and cervical cancer, and verification that HPV tests are performing within proposed guidelines for HPV test performance (Meijer et al. 2009; Booth et al. 2013).

Workload Limits

An important component of any cytology quality program includes provisions for setting up and monitoring the maximum workload (described in terms of slides per hour) for individual cytotechnologists. Federal law in the USA requires that cytotechnologists manually document the number of slides screened within each 24-h period, and the number of hours they spend screening slides each day. This includes slides rescreened for QC purposes. Guidelines prohibit screening more than 100 conventional Pap smear slides, or (per current FDA workload limits for automated image-assisted screening methods) 170 slides/day for the FocalPoint GS and 200 slides/day for the ThinPrep Imaging System over an 8-h period, and not more than 12.5 slides per hour. This also applies to pathologists who perform primary screening. Higher limits are permissible when screening Pap tests that have been imaged and screened by computer systems, since the cytotechnologist reviews a smaller surface area microscopically. All liquid-based Pap test slides with field of view (FOV) only review count as half (0.5) slides, but if they also undergo subsequent manual review they count as 1.5 slides. This is true for new slides and rescreened slides. However, available data based on 100 % rescreening now indicate that screening over 100 slides per day with automated screening devices is associated with substandard screening sensitivity and should not be done. Considerably lower screening rates are associated with highest screening sensitivities (Elsheikh et al. 2010; Levi et al. 2012). Evidence-based recommendations of the American Society of Cytopathology (ASC) task force published in 2013 propose that for gynecologic

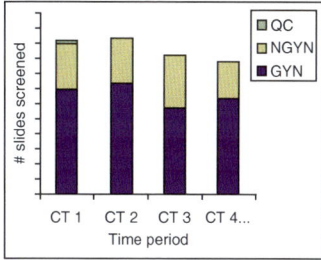 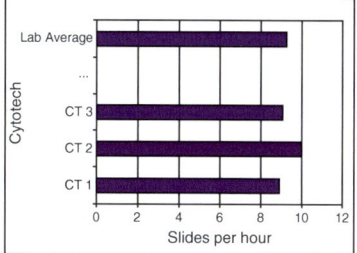

FIG. 9.3 Graphic representation of (*left*) total slide count by cyto-technologist (CT) and (*right*) slides screened per hour by CT (image courtesy of Dr. Robert Goulart, Springfield, MA, USA)

specimens with image-assisted screening the average labora-tory cytotechnologist workload should not exceed 70 slides/day (Elsheikh et al. 2013). When counting slides for work-load, non-gynecologic slides (e.g., exfoliative slides) prepared by a liquid-based or concentration method (ThinPrep, SurePath, or Cytospin), as well as cell block sections, can be counted as half slides. A cellular FNA smear that covers more than half of the slide counts as a full slide. The LIS is often leveraged to keep track of these metrics, and lock out individual cytotechnologists once their case limits have been reached (Fig. 9.3).

Performance Measures

Many labs utilize indicators (e.g., false negative rates, intral-aboratory comparisons) as an objective measure of an indi-vidual's "competency" performance. Data from the LIS is typically analyzed for this purpose. Screening skills of a cytotechnologist can be evaluated by monitoring their abnor-mal rate and false negative cases (detected via 10 % rescreen-ing). Interpretive skills can also be gleaned by monitoring cytotechnologist statistics (e.g., abnormal or pickup rate, unsatisfactory rate) compared with laboratory statistics, by

TABLE 9.4 Contingency table for deriving Pap test metrics

Pap test result	Surgical biopsy result		Metric
	Positive	**Negative**	**Metric**
Positive	True positive (TP)	False positive (FP)	PPV (=TP/TP + FP)
Negative	False negative (FN)	True negative (TN)	NPV (TN/TN + FN))
Metric	Sensitivity (=TP/TP + FN)	Specificity (=TN/TN + FP)	

NPV negative predictive value, *PPV* positive predictive value

keeping a cytotechnologist–cytopathologist discrepancy log for cases submitted to pathologists for review, as well as tracking their performance on proficiency tests. The abnormal rate for a cytotechnologist = their abnormal cases (ASC, AGC, SIL, AIS, carcinoma)/their total cases. This rate can be compared with the lab average. Rates below the average imply that abnormal cases are being missed. False negative Pap tests (Table 9.4) are largely due to sampling error (i.e., lesional cells were not effectively collected and transferred to the glass slide), and are infrequently caused by a lab error (e.g., abnormal cells were missed during screening, or misinterpreted as benign). These metrics are not ideal, since patients with negative Pap test results usually do not get biopsied.

Computer Software

In laboratories where thousands of Pap tests are received, screened and reported, capturing and analyzing QA data can only be accomplished using the LIS. This is sometimes limiting for labs because not all of the information in the LIS is stored as discrete data. In such cases natural language searches may need to be run. Moreover, the LIS often only permits a limited number of QA-related reports to be run, and has inadequate tools to perform sophisticated data manipulation, analysis, and presentation. As a result, cytology QA often involves extracting data from the LIS into external programs (e.g., Microsoft Excel or Access). LIS data retrieval and manipulation is therefore a critical aspect of effective QA.

Both Excel and Access can be used to conduct queries, sort and filter data, merge datasets, run calculations, make pivot tables/charts to more easily view data, and generate reports. Excel is adequate to organize non-relational (or flat) data into worksheets, in rows and columns of cells. However, when dealing with a very large amount of data (thousands of entries), or when there is a need to store data in more than one table and to perform complex queries of these different tables (relational database), then a database management system such as Access is better. Access stores data in tables, but with columns and records (not rows). For most cytology laboratories, Microsoft Excel will be the program of choice to calculate efficiency and error metrics due to its relative simplicity. Currently, Excel will permit the usage of over one million rows of data, which should be sufficient to analyze most cytology operations. An alternative solution to performing QA is to employ middleware with business intelligence platforms (e.g., Altosoft). These applications can help automatically extract LIS data for analysis, and often make it easier to manipulate and combine data from other information systems.

All QA data saved outside of the LIS needs to be secure and protected. This involves creating backup copies of files each time data is updated, using "show/hide" options to remove critical data from view where possible, and limiting user access to this data (e.g., user-level permissions, password requirements, read-only privileges, and encryption).

Excel Spreadsheets

Basic spreadsheets permit users great flexibility in terms of data manipulation. Table 9.5 highlights some helpful Excel formulas. Spreadsheets offer a dynamic quality to the data, as

TABLE 9.5 Common and useful excel formulas

=**NETWORKDAYS** () This formula returns the total number of whole workdays between two dates. This count excludes weekends. For instance, if the lab in question has a weekday operation, using the formula = NETWORKDAYS () and referencing the accession and signout date in the formula will return the number of workdays it took to complete a case

=**Days360** () This formula returns the number of days between two dates based on a 360 day calendar. This count includes weekends. For instance, if the lab in question is a 24/7 operation, using the formula = DAYS360 () and referencing the accession and signout date in the formula will return the number of days it took to complete the case

=**Vlookup** () This formula looks for the value in the left most column of a table and returns the value in the same row from which you specify, from a different table. The data, however, must be sorted in ascending order. This formula is very useful because very often a single report (dataset) from the LIS will not supply all of the information needed. This helps simplify combining two or more datasets into a single spreadsheet that is more useful. Typically, a case number is an ideal value to use as an association between two reports

---

data can be charted, sorted, and organized into tables. The basic types of data that can be entered into a spreadsheet are text (with no numerical value), constants (a number), and formulas. Most laboratory software solutions accommodate the downloading of data into spreadsheets. For those labs that cannot save their LIS data directly into an Excel file, but can save it as a text file (*.txt, *.csv, etc.; where csv = comma separated value), the text import wizard is highly useful and is a three step process:

- *Step 1.* The first screen appears once the file is selected (Fig. 9.4). Since the data being saved is in table format, the selection of delimited is ideal.
- *Step 2.* The next window (Fig. 9.5) allows the user to determine how they would like the data separated. The most common selections are Comma separated or Tab separated.

- *Step 3.* The last window of the three window series (Fig. 9.6) allows modification to the column data format, the default of "General" is typically correct.

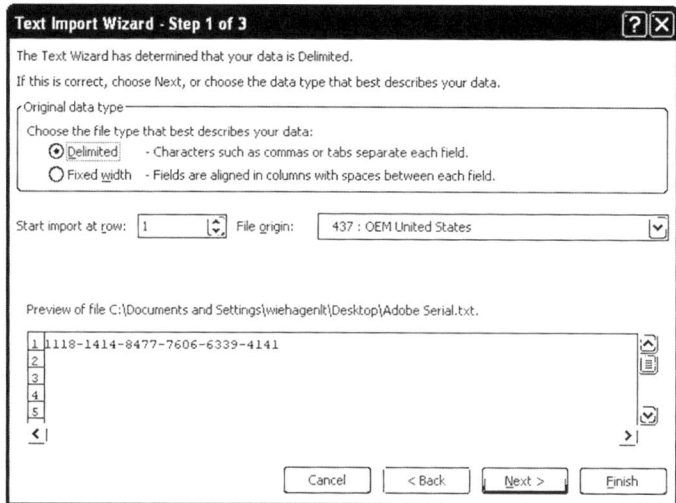

Text Import Wizard - Step 1 of 3

The Text Wizard has determined that your data is Delimited.

If this is correct, choose Next, or choose the data type that best describes your data.

Original data type

Choose the file type that best describes your data:
- ⦿ Delimited   - Characters such as commas or tabs separate each field.
- ○ Fixed width   - Fields are aligned in columns with spaces between each field.

Start import at row: 1   File origin: 437 : OEM United States

Preview of file C:\Documents and Settings\wiehagenlt\Desktop\Adobe Serial.txt.

1 1118-1414-8477-7606-6339-4141
2
3
4
5

Cancel   < Back   Next >   Finish

FIG. 9.4 **Step 1 of 3** provides options (delimited or fixed width) on the type of data being imported into Excel. Delimited data is separated by a character and fixed width data implies that the data is standardized across all fields (LIS data is rarely stored in a fixed width manner)

Pivot Tables

Pivot tables are highly useful to summarize large data sets. These are dynamic tables that allow data to be summarized in different ways without the need for a formula. They are particularly useful when analyzing relationships between data points. For instance, in Fig. 9.7 this simple data table has five columns used to calculate turnaround time. By utilizing the Pivot Table Field List (Fig. 9.8) you can simply drag and drop the column headings into the appropriate area for sorting. When using pivot tables, identification of the columns of data in your table is important. Therefore, depending on the labels applied by the LIS, relabeling the columns may make them more easily identified.

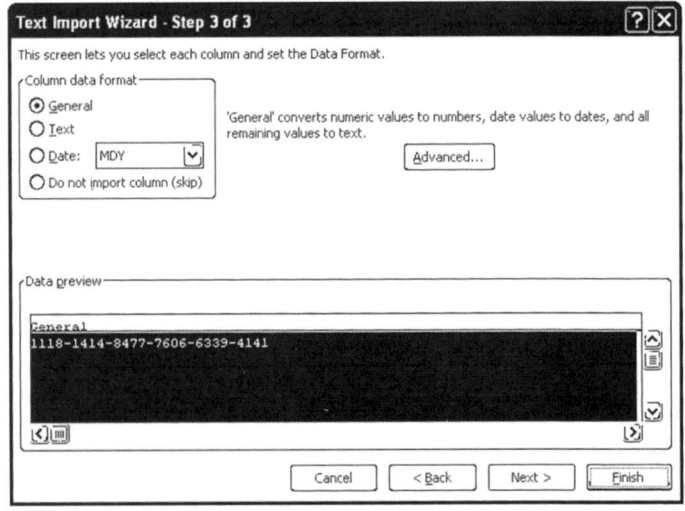

Text Import Wizard - Step 2 of 3

This screen lets you set the delimiters your data contains. You can see how your text is affected in the preview below.

Delimiters
- ☑ Tab
- ☐ Semicolon
- ☐ Comma
- ☐ Space
- ☐ Other:

☐ Treat consecutive delimiters as one

Text qualifier: "

Data preview

1118-1414-8477-7606-6339-4141

Cancel < Back Next > Finish

FIG. 9.5 Step 2 of 3 provides options (delimiters) for defining the manner in which the data being imported is delimitated. By default the Tab option is selected. However, if the file is saved as a *.CSV, then the comma section should be selected

Text Import Wizard - Step 3 of 3

This screen lets you select each column and set the Data Format.

Column data format
- ⦿ General
- ○ Text
- ○ Date: MDY
- ○ Do not import column (skip)

'General' converts numeric values to numbers, date values to dates, and all remaining values to text.

Advanced...

Data preview

General
1118-1414-8477-7606-6339-4141

Cancel < Back Next > Finish

FIG. 9.6 Step 3 of 3 provides a preview of the data import and options for further defining the data

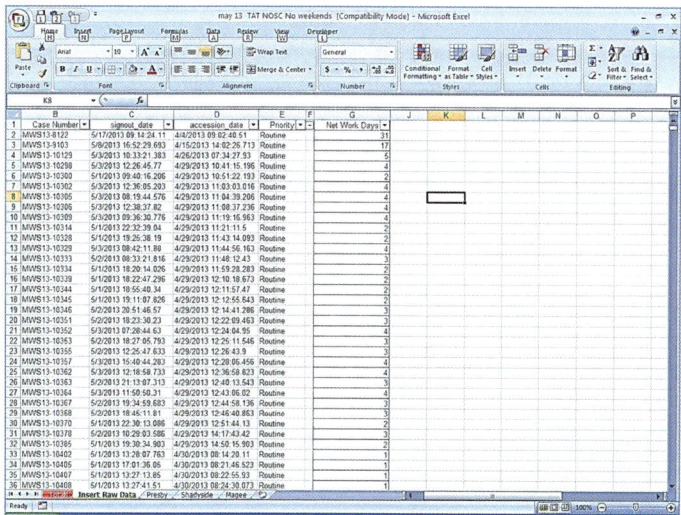

FIG. 9.7 Tabulated data with five columns (de-identified case number, signout date, accession date, priority and network days/turnaround time)

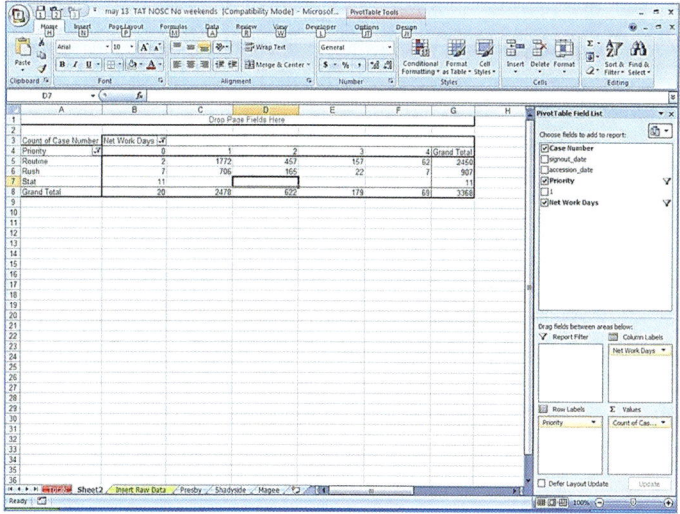

FIG. 9.8 Shows the pivot table of the example in Fig. 9.7 with a count of cases signed out by priority after 0–4 days

References

Austin RM, Zhao C. Observations on Pap test litigation. Pathol Case Rev. 2011;16:73–82.

Booth CN, Bashleben C, Filomena CA, et al. Monitoring and ordering practices for human papillomavirus in cervical cytology findings from the College of American Pathologists gynecologic cytopathology quality consensus conference working group 5. Arch Path Lab Med. 2013;137:214–9.

Cibas ES, Zou KH, Crum CP, et al. Using the rate of positive high-risk HPV test results for ASCUS together with the ASCUS/SIL ratio in evaluating the performance of cytopathologists. Am J Clin Pathol. 2008;129:97–101.

Clary KM, Davey DD, Naryshkin S, Austin RM, Chmara BA, Tworek J. The role of monitoring interpretive rates, concordance between cytotechnologist and pathologist interpretations prior to sign-out, and turn-around-time in gynecologic quality assurance: findings from the College of American Pathologists gynecologic cytopathology quality consensus conference. Working group 1. Arch Pathol Lab Med. 2013;137:164–74.

Elsheikh TM, Kirkpatrick JL, Cooper MK, Johnson ML, Hawkins AP, Rernshaw AA. Increasing cytotechnologist workload above 100 slides per day using the ThinPrep Imaging System leads to significant reductions in screening accuracy. Cancer Cytopathol. 2010;118:75–82.

Elsheikh TM, Austin RM, Chhieng DF, Miller FS, Moriarty AT, Renshaw AA, American Society of Cytopathology. American Society of Cytopathology workload recommendations for automated Pap test screening: developed by the productivity and quality assurance in the era of automated screening task force. Diagn Cytopathol. 2013;41:174–8.

Eversole GM, Moriarty AT, Schwartz MR, et al. Practices of participants in the College of American Pathologists interlaboratory comparison program in cervicovaginal cytology. Arch Pathol Lab Med. 2010;134:331–5.

Levi AW, Galullo P, Gordy K, Mikolaiski, et al. Increasing cytotechnologist workload above 100 slides per day using BD FocalPoint GS Imaging System negatively affects screening performance. Am J Clin Pathol. 2012;138:811–5.

Meijer CM, Berkhof JB, Castle PE, et al. Guidelines for human papillomavirus DNA test requirements for primary cervical cancer screening in women 30 years and older. Int J Cancer. 2009;124:516–20.

Renshaw A, Deschene M, Auger M. ASC/SIL ratio for cytotechnologists. A surrogate marker of screening sensitivity. Am J Clin Pathol. 2009;131:776–8.

Tavares SB, de Sousa NL, Manrique EJ, et al. Rapid pre-screening of cervical smears as a method of internal quality control in a cervical screening programme. Cytopathology. 2008;19:254–9.

Tworek JA, Jones BA, Raab S, Clary KM, Walsh M. The value of monitoring human papillomavirus DNA results for Papanicolaou tests diagnosed as atypical squamous cells of undetermined significance. A College of American Pathologists Q-Probes study of 68 institutions. Arch Pathol Lab Med. 2007;131:1525–31.

Zhao C, Florea A, Onisko A, Austin RM. Histologic follow-up results in 662 patients with Pap test findings of atypical glandular cells: results from a large academic women's hospital laboratory employing sensitive screening methods. Gynecol Oncol. 2009;114:383–9.

Chapter 10
Barcoding

Ioan C. Cucoranu, Anil V. Parwani, and Liron Pantanowitz

Introduction

In cytology there are many physical assets that need to be identified and sometimes tracked. These assets include paper requisitions, specimen containers, cassettes (cell blocks, core biopsies), glass slides, and other materials (e.g., reagent inventories). This becomes complicated when these assets need to be shared with other divisions of the laboratory (e.g., aliquoting of a fluid sample for flow cytometry or microbiology testing). This process was traditionally performed manually using written logs. However, tracking has improved and has become more automated with newer laboratory information systems (LIS), middleware, and the use of technology such as barcodes and radio-frequency identification (RFID) tags.

I.C. Cucoranu, M.D. (✉) • A.V. Parwani, M.D., Ph.D., M.B.A.
L. Pantanowitz, M.D.
Department of Pathology, University of Pittsburgh Medical Center, Pittsburgh, PA, USA
e-mail: cucoranuic@upmc.edu; parwaniav@upmc.edu; pantanowitzl@upmc.edu

L. Pantanowitz and A.V. Parwani (eds.), *Practical Informatics for Cytopathology*, Essentials in Cytopathology 14, DOI 10.1007/978-1-4614-9581-9_10,
© Springer Science+Business Media New York 2014

There are several good reasons to implement tracking. The first is to be able to track the identification, status and/or location of a unique item (i.e., asset management or traceability). Tracking can also help maximize workflow efficiency (e.g., promotes Lean methods, just-in-time techniques, and automation). This is becoming increasingly important with the demands for faster turnaround times in the face of increasing test volumes, fewer staff, and greater complexity (e.g., need to perform ancillary tests). Tracking also permits laboratories to detect workflow bottlenecks, often in real-time. Using barcode driven protocols helps guide and standardize workflow. Adverse patient events may occur because of misidentification or labeling errors in the laboratory. This is often the result of staff manually labeling items, illegible handwriting, batch-match tasks, and use of shortcuts (so-called "work-arounds") that circumvents standard protocol. Improperly identified specimens may cause a delay in diagnosis, unnecessary additional investigations or testing which are sometimes invasive, and in the most extreme circumstances treatment of the wrong patient for the wrong disease. Identification errors can be reduced by adopting positive patient identification (PPID), i.e., correct identification of a patient and linking of all specimens to that patient. Automatically capturing data with a barcode scanner directly into the LIS is more accurate than manual key entry. This helps minimize identification errors and thereby promotes patient safety and reduces medical–legal liability. Since tracking data is being captured in the LIS, this measurable data can be used for metrics as part of an overall quality assurance (QA) program.

Barcode Systems

A barcode is an optically machine readable representation of data using characters represented by patterns. There are 1D and 2D barcode symbologies (Fig. 10.1). Linear (1D) barcodes may include numerical (e.g., Codabar, UPC) or alphanumerical

Fɪɢ. 10.1 Examples of 1D and 2D barcode symbologies for the statement "Cytology 2013." The quick response (QR) barcode shown on the *right* is a matrix of *black* modules (*square dots*) arranged in a grid

(e.g., code 128) data. 2D barcodes (e.g., DataMatrix, MaxiCode, QR code) are smaller (require smaller labels), permit higher data density, are scalable, allow omnidirectional scanning, and have fewer scan and printer failures. Although complete standardization of barcodes in the clinical laboratory remains to be achieved, such efforts are underway, including the AUTO-12A barcode label standard issued by the Clinical Laboratory Standards Institute (CLSI). Apart from barcodes, other label parameters that are important include their size, space for additional readable data/text (e.g., patient name, accession number, stain type), font, and color. Some colors (e.g., dark colors or red, aqua, and blue) may make it hard to read barcodes. Barcode scanners act as "keyboard data input" by transferring the information encoded in barcodes directly into the LIS (Fig. 10.2).

Radio-Frequency Identification

RFID tags are small transponders that use radio-frequency signals. When affixed to an asset, they can store unique data about that asset. There are both active and passive RFID tags

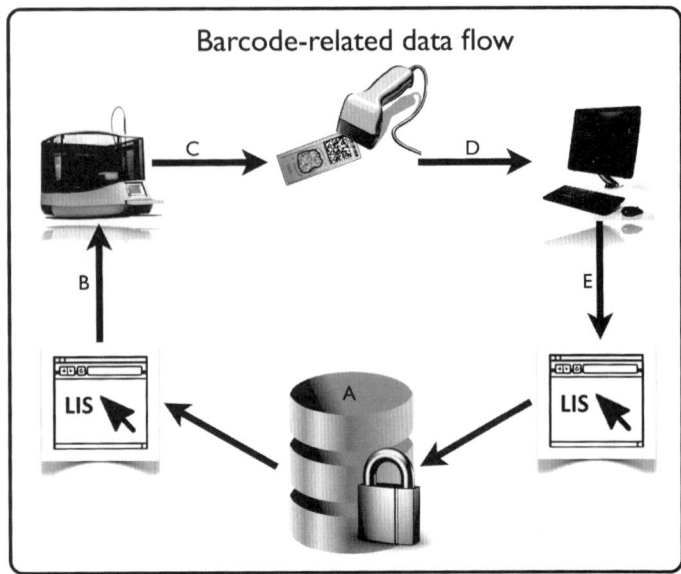

Fig. 10.2 Flow of data in the laboratory information system (LIS) using barcoding. (**a**) A barcode with a unique identification number is linked to patient information in the LIS. Some labs purchase printed barcodes whereas others print them from the LIS in the lab. (**b**) Lab instruments have an internal barcode reader that scans the slide barcode. (**c**) Scanning this encoded barcode present on a glass slide label (**d**) automatically links this asset (glass slide) to the correct patient's case and directly inputs data (e.g., time and location of scanning) into the LIS (**e**)

(Fig. 10.3). RFID technology is being used in limited instances in the anatomical pathology lab (e.g., with specimen couriers). While RFID tags are more rugged (i.e., they exhibit a near flawless read rate), have greater capacity to store data, allow data to be updated if needed, and are easier to read (e.g., up to 1,000 tags can be simultaneously read) when compared to barcodes, they are currently more expensive.

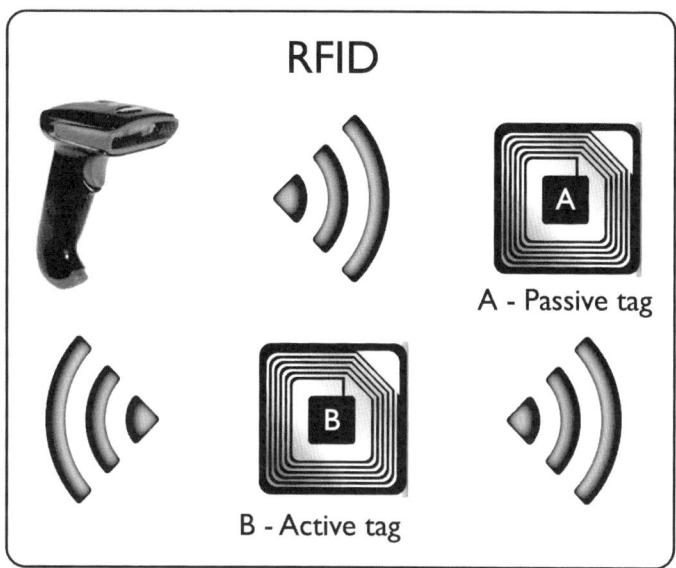

Fig. 10.3 RFID tags. (*Top*) A passive tag only transmits data (chirps) when scanned by a reader. (*Bottom*) An active tag has its own power source and continuously broadcasts a signal

Barcoding Technology

Software

Software used for tracking may be integrated within a LIS (e.g., tracking module) or installed as separate middleware (e.g., Vantage, Cerebro, OmniTrax, CheckMate, and HTS from General Data). Either software solution needs to demonstrate interoperability with the cytology lab's instruments. However, there are some middleware solutions and instruments that unfortunately use their own proprietary barcoding systems, which may therefore be incompatible with other tracking solutions. In such cases, laboratories may need to use two different barcodes on their assets. The ideal tracking software should be flexible (e.g., easy to configure), user friendly, and suitable for a range of platforms (e.g., desktop computers, touch screens, handheld devices).

Hardware

Hardware for tracking includes computers, bar code readers and printers. These devices will need to be placed where scanning of barcodes is required (e.g., microtomy workstations). When implementing a system in the laboratory it is important to pay attention to the footprint, durability, and software compatibility of these devices.

- *Barcode readers*. Available barcode scanners include contact wands, scanners with laser triggers, and readers that contain a charge coupled device (CCD). These scanners can be wireless or wired. Some barcode readers may only be able to read 1D barcodes, while others may be backwards compatible and can read both 1D and 2D formats.
- *Label printers*. Printers that use thermal technology are more desirable, because labels will need to withstand harsh environments (e.g., chemicals like xylene, heat, and microwave processing). Durable labels will hopefully not wash off, erase, or darken.
- *Cassette printers*. These instruments can have a single hopper (one magazine to hold cassettes) or multiple hoppers (e.g., 1–12 magazines that hold cassettes with different colors) (Fig. 10.4).
- *Slide printers*. There are slide printers that print labels that are later affixed to slides, print directly onto slides, or laser etch barcodes directly onto glass slides.

Tracking and Workflow

Workflow in the cytology lab begins with specimen collection. However, not too many laboratories can track specimens at the time of procurement (e.g., when a Pap smear is obtained). For

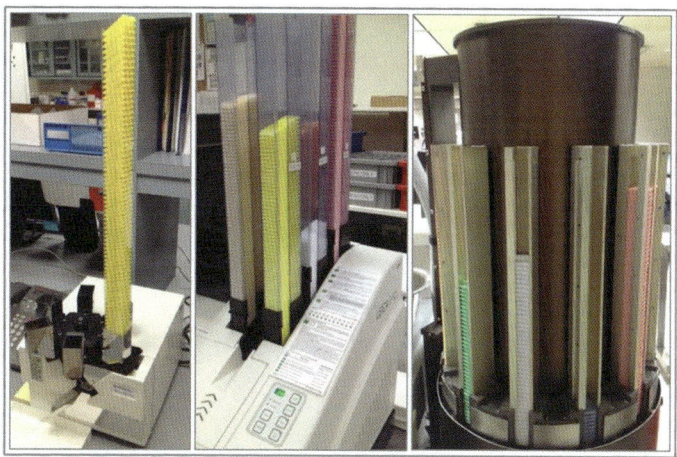

Fig. 10.4 Different cassette printers. The *left panel* shows a printer with one hopper. The *middle panel* shows a printer with multiple magazines and the *right panel* an instrument with a much bigger footprint

tracking to start at the "bedside" the LIS needs to be interfaced with the electronic medical record (EMR). Therefore, when an electronic order is entered in the EMR barcodes generated by the LIS can be printed remotely or pre-printed and then applied to the specimen at pick-up. Such "pre-accessioned" cases remain inactive in the LIS until they reach the lab where they get accessioned. Handheld tracking devices can be used to track outreach specimen vials by couriers. Accessioning occurs when the specimen arrives in the laboratory. If these specimens do not have a barcode on them that is recognized by the LIS, lab staff will need to print and label them (Fig. 10.5). Cassettes with printed barcodes on them may be required if cell blocks are being prepared. While it is important that cassette printers make cassettes just-in-time (JIT) when needed, to avoid errors (from pre-printing,

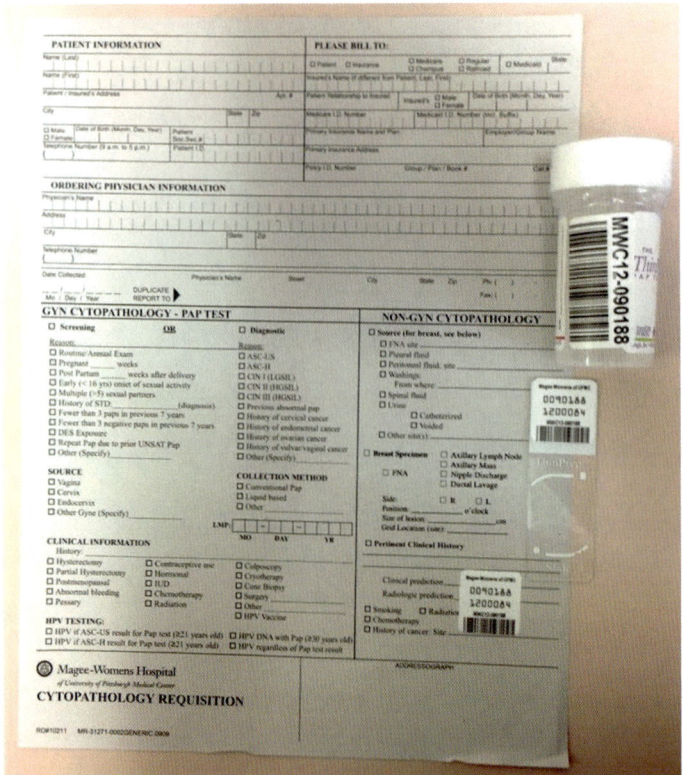

FIG. 10.5 For a given case, labels with the same barcode get affixed to the paper requisition, specimen vial, and in this case the glass slide. (Image courtesy of Joseph Beere, Pittsburgh, PA)

sorting, and distribution), they should still be able to print on-demand and handle batch printing.

Slide identification (ID) procedures may differ depending on the equipment being used in the cytology lab. For example, glass slides prepared on a ThinPrep® 2000 Processor do not use barcodes, so any barcode can be used on the slide by the lab. However, glass slides prepared on a ThinPrep® 3000 Processor for Pap tests or ThinPrep® 5000 Processor for non-gynecological cases do interact with barcodes. The ThinPrep® 3000 reads a 1D barcode on the vial and prints (etches) the corresponding 14 digit Optical Character Recognition (OCR) number on the slide. The ThinPrep® 5000

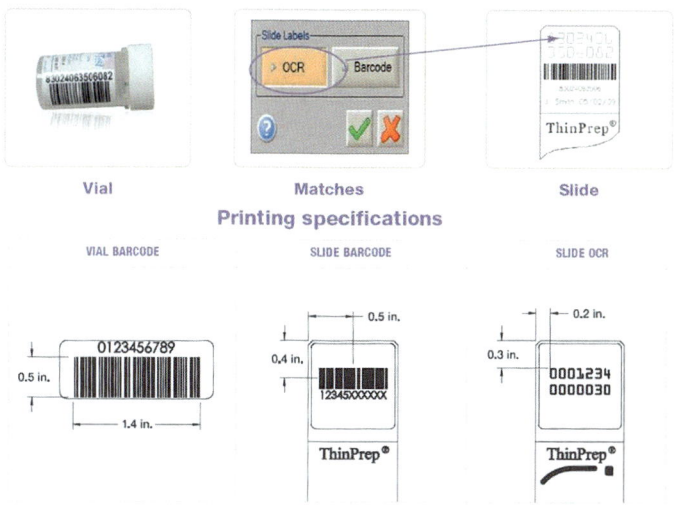

Fig. 10.6 Labeling considerations are shown in the *top panel* for the ThinPrep® 5000 Processor. This instrument can read 1D barcodes or optical character recognition (OCR) on the slide. Printing specifications for vials and slides are shown in the *lower panel* (courtesy of Hologic, Inc. and affiliates)

Processor can read 1D barcodes from the vial, and matches either a 1D or 2D barcode, or 14 digit code on the slide. If a cytology lab uses the PrepStain processing instrument that makes SurePath® slides, hand-held barcode readers may be used to scan the centrifuge tube and corresponding slide on the slide tray to confirm chain of custody. A poor quality barcode or one that is placed in the wrong position may cause this slide to be rejected by a lab instrument. Therefore, it is important to follow the labeling instructions and printing specifications provided by the vendor (Fig. 10.6).

It is important that workstations in the cytology lab have adequate space for barcoding devices, and that they have network access. Access to computer keyboards and monitors in the lab should also be ergonomically situated. Computer screens mounted on mobile arms and touch screen monitors are available for this purpose. Although the cytology lab may submit cell blocks (and sometimes core tissue biopsies) to histology for further processing, details regarding tracking in

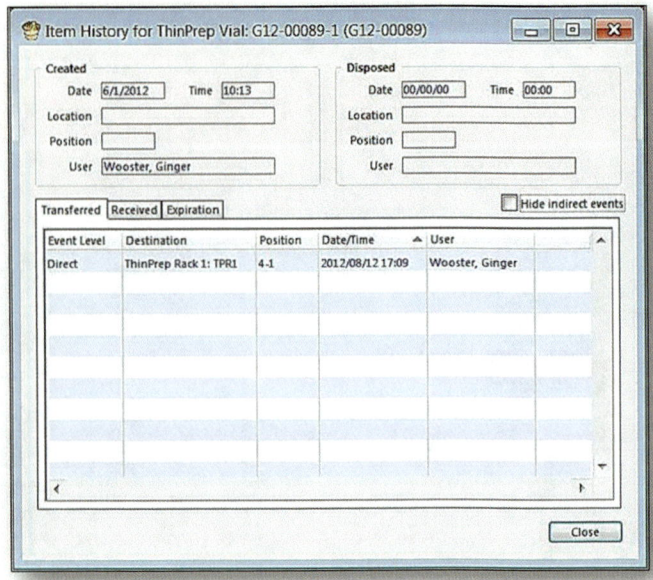

F‌IG. 10.7 The screenshot from this LIS shows how easy it is to retrieve a stored Pap test vial to send for HPV testing. With one click the user knows exactly where (i.e., Rack #1) to locate the vial for this case (image courtesy of Orchard Software, Carmel, Indiana)

the histology lab are beyond the scope of this chapter. Nevertheless, it is important to be aware that most handling and barcoding of assets (blocks and slides) in the histology lab occurs at the microtomy workstation. Once glass slides are prepared and labeled, barcoding can be used to help avoid errors with case assembly (e.g., matching slides with printed working drafts) and to track their delivery.

The last step in this process involves storage and retrieval of specimen vials, slides, and blocks. Retrieval of specimens (e.g., Pap test vials for add-on HPV tests) can be time consuming. Tracking solutions can facilitate quick and easy retrieval of assets, as well as provide accurate documentation of these events in the LIS. Some tracking solutions offer virtual trays/racks for stored vials that can greatly improve locating specimens (Fig. 10.7).

Status Monitors

Labs may want to use a status monitor to view their tracked assets to see if there are any problems or bottlenecks. These dashboards are usually in the form of tables or a spreadsheet. They allow staff to view at-a-glance various activities in the lab, such as the status of all stains (Fig. 10.8). Colors are typically used for this purpose; for example, red is used to alert staff about a potential problem. Labs may opt to have these dashboards displayed on large mounted TV screens or made Web-accessible.

Implementation

Prior to implementation it is important to understand exactly what the lab is trying to accomplish with a tracking solution, e.g., tracking assets, operational efficiency, and/or patient safety. Planning is important (e.g., analysis of existing workflow, designing labels), as is making sure that there are adequate resources available (e.g., IT support, finances for

	Ordered	Labeled	Stained	Delivered	Missing
Routine	543	2765	45	134	-
IHC stains	45	34	15	12	-
Specials	24	55	4	-	-
Cell blocks	13	3	16	-	4
Others	57	392	7	8	-

FIG. 10.8 Example of a stain status monitor. *Green fields* indicate that those stains in the process are proceeding without delay. *Yellow* indicates that there is an acceptable delay. *Red* in this example alerts the lab that there are 4 cell block slides missing

hidden costs like vendor consultation). The lab infrastructure will need to accommodate this new technology (e.g., adequate space, wiring, network drops). Trying out equipment in the lab before purchasing will help avoid pitfalls later. Interoperability with the LIS and instrument interfaces is essential. Although vendor tracking solutions today are fairly sophisticated, they will still require some configuration (customization). It is advisable for the cytology lab to work closely with their vendor representative to determine the right label placement, barcode symbology to use, and other specifications before deciding on barcoding altogether. This can simplify the process if these issues are discussed up front. Trying to get a legacy barcode to work may be more challenging than starting with the right specifications from the beginning. Finally, in order for any tracking solution to be successful there will need to have buy-in from all staff involved as well as leadership. It is important to realize that jobs will change, staff will initially need to overcome a learning curve, and that ongoing compliance is crucial.

Chapter 11
Informatics Projects

Liron Pantanowitz

Introduction

A project refers to a temporary effort with established goals that need to be achieved. They differ from operations which are the routine, ongoing, and repetitive business processes in the laboratory. There are usually several informatics projects ongoing or planned in a pathology laboratory. These may directly or indirectly impact cytopathology, given that informatics plays a pivotal role in all areas of the lab. Therefore, it is important that cytologists are aware of the information technology (IT) project life cycle and some broad issues related to project management in informatics.

L. Pantanowitz, M.D. (✉)
Department of Pathology, University of Pittsburgh Medical Center,
Pittsburgh, PA, USA
e-mail: pantanowtizl@upmc.edu

L. Pantanowitz and A.V. Parwani (eds.), *Practical Informatics*
for Cytopathology, Essentials in Cytopathology 14,
DOI 10.1007/978-1-4614-9581-9_11,
© Springer Science+Business Media New York 2014

Project Life Cycle

Like most projects, informatics projects develop over five phases. These include the (1) initiating (conceptual) phase, (2) the planning phase, (3) the executing phase, and (4) the controlling (monitoring) phase, followed by (5) the closing (completion) phase of a project (Fig. 11.1). These phases may overlap throughout a project. Also, some projects may be terminated before they reach completion and others may go through these steps more than once. Sometimes a project charter may be used to outline the purpose, scope, and other parameters of a project. This document may also provide details about the project plan, implementation, and specific deliverables. The controlling step should not be avoided, because when project performance is regularly observed and measured, problems can be identified early and speedily acted on. The closing phase of a project involves not only preparing the lab to take over operations (e.g., training, trans- ferring responsibilities), but is also used to assess success, reward the project team, and record any lessons learned that may be helpful on future projects.

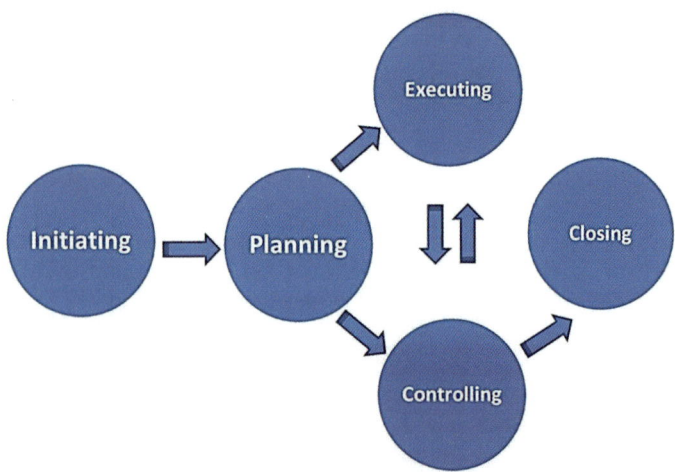

Fig. 11.1 Development phases of a project

Project Management

Projects are judged to be successful based on whether their goals were achieved within the desired budget, timetable and completed with the intended level of quality. Projects may fail if they are not well planned and/or executed. Effective project management can help reduce the stress for those individuals involved or that may be impacted by projects. It can also reduce costs and improve quality. A major challenge of project management is to balance quality, scope, time, and the cost involved in a project (Fig. 11.2). At the outset, it is valuable to establish a set scope (i.e., what is included, and what is not included). Otherwise, "mission creep" may delay completion of the project. Time management is critical and involves establishing and meeting deadlines, but also dealing with slippage. Management of finances (budgets and cash flow) may require a trade off with other competing elements such as time and quality. Effective management also involves good communication with all stakeholders (e.g., team members, clients, vendors) and ably dealing with people (e.g., motivation, running meetings, conflict resolution). The

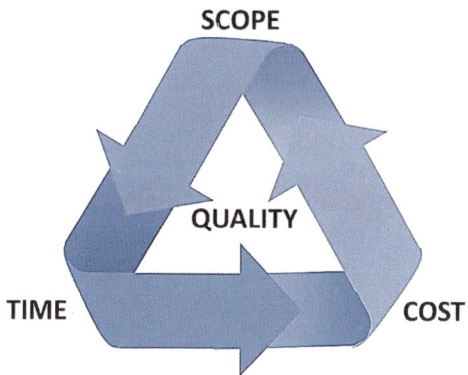

FIG. 11.2 Project management triangle. It should be evident that one side (a project constraint) of the triangle cannot be changed without affecting the others

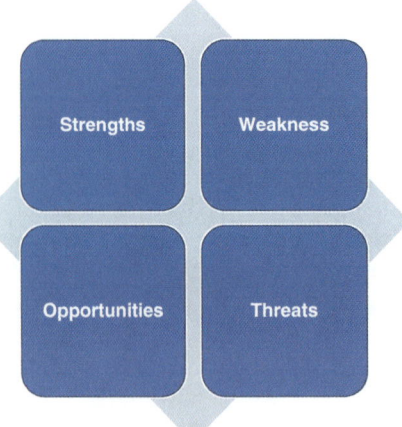

Fig. 11.3 SWOT analysis

informaticist plays a key role in coordinating projects, and helps make sure that everything comes together. Unfortunately, everything doesn't always work out as planned. Hence, it is important to be able to also manage risks (e.g., technological, financial, legal, and managerial risk).

Business Strategy

Informatics helps organizations achieve their business mission. Therefore, informatics tools and projects are important when it comes to an organization's overall strategy. In the clinical laboratory, pathology leadership and laboratory managers are key players in helping an organization achieve their vision. They may be called upon to help make certain strategic decisions. There are several validated techniques available to assist with decision making, one of which is the SWOT (Strengths, Weaknesses, Opportunities, and Threats) analysis (Fig. 11.3). This simple method can help the lab understand the important factors (internal and external) to anticipate when making a decision. The strength of this technique is that it maintains a broad focus during the decision-making process, so that key factors are not left out of consideration. The SWOT technique also balances an idealistic outlook with consideration of what can go wrong, and prevents negative thinking from overlooking opportunities or strengths.

Chapter 12
Lean Six Sigma

Ioan C. Cucoranu, Anil V. Parwani, and Liron Pantanowitz

Introduction

Since the 1999 report entitled *To Err is Human* from the Institute of Medicine (IOM) about the high rate of medical errors, there have been many measures to improve patient safety and reduce errors in healthcare. Many cytology laboratories have accordingly adopted *Lean Six Sigma* tools to help improve quality, reduce potential errors, and enhance business efficiency (Table 12.1). To reap the benefits of these toolkits for their laboratories, cytologists need to have some understanding of these manufacturing industry concepts. The key principles of combining Lean and Six Sigma strategies are summarized in Table 12.2. Informatics plays a key role in implementing and supporting these tools (e.g., computers, automation).

I.C. Cucoranu, M.D. (✉) • A.V. Parwani, M.D., Ph.D., M.B.A.
L. Pantanowitz, M.D.
Department of Pathology, University of Pittsburgh Medical Center, Pittsburgh, PA, USA
e-mail: cucoranuic@upmc.edu; parwaniav@upmc.edu; pantanowitzl@upmc.edu

L. Pantanowitz and A.V. Parwani (eds.), *Practical Informatics for Cytopathology*, Essentials in Cytopathology 14, DOI 10.1007/978-1-4614-9581-9_12,
© Springer Science+Business Media New York 2014

TABLE 12.1 Lean Six Sigma management approaches

Concept	Explanation
Lean	A culture using tools aimed at minimizing waste and creating more value while doing less work
Six Sigma	A data-driven approach to error reduction by improving processes and reducing process variability

TABLE 12.2 Key principles of Lean Six Sigma

- Focus on the customer (i.e., the patient and/or physician)
- Identify and understand how work in the lab gets done (the value stream)
- Manage, improve and make workflow more efficient
- Remove non-value-added steps and waste
- Manage the lab using data and reduce workflow variation
- Empower (involve and equip) the people in the process
- Systematically undertake improvements in all activities

Toyota Production System

The Toyota Production System (TPS) is an integrated, socio-technical system developed by Toyota for their automobile manufacturing. *The Toyota Way* comprises management philosophy and practices directed towards organizing manufacturing and logistics, including the interaction with suppliers and customers. TPS is a precursor of the Lean manufacturing system. The two main principles of TPS are continuous improvement (e.g., innovation) and respect for people (e.g., teamwork) (Fig. 12.1). With the TPS there are defined work rules that focus on standardized workflow. Under the guidance of a team leader, the principle is to continuously improve the quality of products and services. This can be achieved by continuously redesigning processes in order to

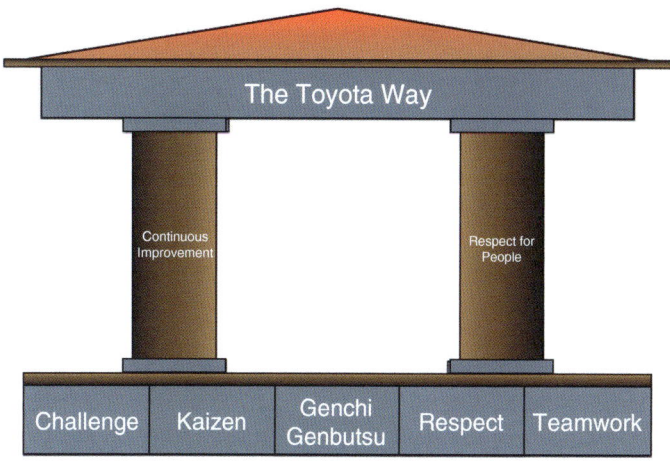

Fig. 12.1 Model of *The Toyota Way*. The two main pillars are Continuous Improvement and Respect for People. *Challenge* refers not only to embracing challenges but also challenging the status quo in order to make changes for improvement. *Kaizen* refers to promoting a continuous step-by-step approach for improved performance. *Genchi Genbutsu* literally means "going to the source," indicating that sound decision-making requires checking the facts first-hand. *Respect* involves respecting not only the individuality of each employee but also their contributions, ideas, and cultural or personal beliefs. *Teamwork* promotes people working together at all levels

eliminate waste. Problems are best identified in real-time, by the individuals performing the work. In order to successfully implement the TPS, leadership needs to encourage and support a worker-empowered culture for continual improvement. This is hard to achieve with a more traditional managerial approach based on sporadic, leader-directed quality assurance (QA) projects. The TPS has proven to be a practical method for standardizing Pap test reporting, FNA immediate adequacy interpretation, and for reducing overall errors in the cytology lab.

Lean Method

Lean tools help reduce waste associated with the flow of materials and information in a process from beginning (e.g., specimen procurement) to end (e.g., report delivery). The goal is to identify and eliminate nonessential and non-value-added steps in the workflow process in order to streamline production, improve quality, and gain customer loyalty. Lean methods augment Six Sigma tools by improving the speed and efficiency of workflow processes. The mnemonic "TIMWOOD" is used to highlight the kinds of waste to be eliminated (Table 12.3). The goal for a cytology laboratory to be Lean is to use less effort, fewer resources, and less time to handle, interpret, and report on incoming samples. To implement Lean a lab needs to exploit the following principles:

- *Specify value*: Identify and categorize those steps in the lab that are "value added" and "non-value added," with the purpose of eliminating or reducing the latter activities.
- *Identify the value stream*: Develop a value stream map of the overall process (i.e., a special flowchart using Lean symbols to depict and improve the flow of inventory and information).
- *Create a "pull" workflow system*: Keep the flow of work in the lab continuously moving in order to avoid queuing (waiting) between steps.
- *Heijunka*: Level the workload and mix of sample types in the lab to improve productivity and/or lead time.
- *Eliminate waste* (*muda*): Develop solutions and reengineer processes to eliminate or reduce any non-value-added tasks.
- *Just in time* (*JIT*) *strategy*: Produce the next part in the testing process, such as a slide or cassette, only when needed. This helps reduce in-process inventory and the potential for identification errors.
- *Manage performance*: Regularly review performance, ensuring that key performance indicators are good and that the overall process is "in control".

TABLE 12.3 Seven types of muda (waste)

Mnemonic	Waste	Examples of waste in the cytology laboratory
T	Transportation	Unnecessary transport of materials (specimens, supplies, FNA microscope carts, slides) and reports
I	Inventory	Excess stock of supplies as well as a disorganized lab, workstations and offices
M	Motion	Poor layout and manual tasks causing wear and tear on equipment and repetitive strain injuries for workers
W	Waiting	Downtime and uneven workflow related to pushed, batched, and extra steps as well as equipment failure
O	Over-processing	Doing extra work, added steps, generating superfluous manual logs, or using unnecessary and expensive tools
O	Over-production	Performing more work such as making too many slides or producing items earlier than needed
D	Defects	Workarounds and rework related to errors, mislabeling, broken equipment, and rescheduling of procedures

Six Sigma

The Six Sigma manufacturing strategy developed by Motorola has been successfully implemented by several companies, most notably General Electric (GE). Six Sigma is based on the concept that defects (errors) and variability in processes (manufacturing) can be reduced by effectively using data and statistical analysis. The ideal goal is to fix a process so that it will be 99.9997 % defect free (six Standard Deviations) or

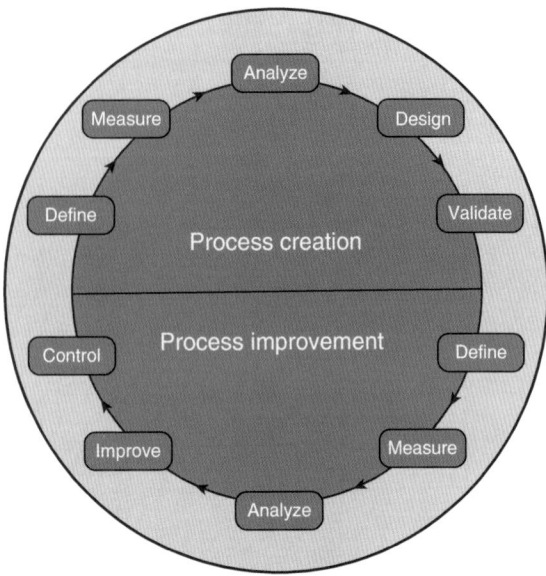

Fig. 12.2 Six-Sigma project methodologies

produce only 3.4 defects per million opportunities (DPMO). For example, for a large cytology laboratory this would mean generating only 3.4 erroneous cytology reports for one million Pap tests processed. Six Sigma projects follow two methodologies, which are DMAIC (Define, Measure, Analyze, Improve, Control) and DMADV (Define, Measure, Analyze, Design, Validate) (Fig. 12.2). DMAIC is used for projects aimed at improving an existing process, while DMADV is used to create a new product or process design. DMAIC begins by defining the problem (project goals), measuring key aspects of the current process (which involves data collection), and then analyzing data (for cause-and-effect relationships, seeking out the root cause of the defect under investigation). Thereafter, a defective process can be improved (or optimized); making sure that there is control of future process to ensure that deviations from target are corrected before they result in defects (e.g., using production boards, visual workplaces, and continuous monitoring).

Unlike Lean philosophy which is a bottom-up process, heavily relying on workers to identify problems, Six Sigma is a leader-driven system.

The Deming Cycle

The Deming cycle is also known as the PDCA (plan–do–check–act) cycle. This four-step management method is used for the control and continuous improvement of many processes and products (Fig. 12.3). The PDCA cycle underlies many Lean operations and is also used in Six Sigma programs (e.g., where the PDCA cycle is called DMAIC). Cytology laboratories can incorporate the PDCA cycle into their quality management program to help with continuous improvement, as well as when implementing any change, starting a new project, for root cause analyses to verify and prioritize problems, designing an improved process, or offering a new product or service.

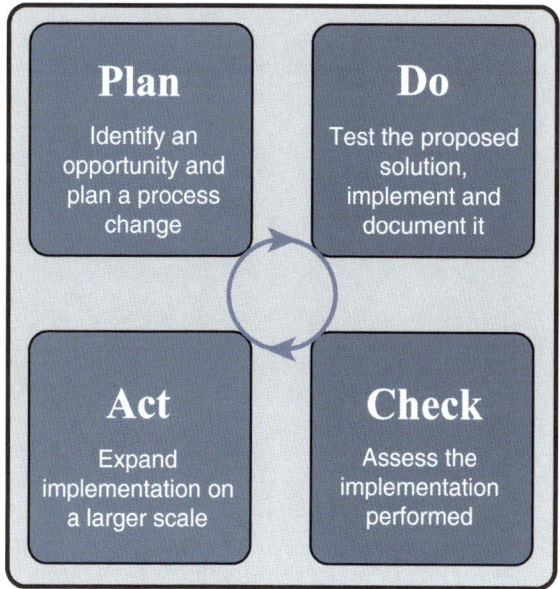

FIG. 12.3 The Deming cycle

Chapter 13
Electronic Medical Records

Seung L. Park, Anil V. Parwani, and Liron Pantanowitz

Introduction

An electronic health record (EHR), also known as an electronic medical record (EMR), is a patient's medical chart accessed and modified in digital format. While an EMR is under the direct control of a hospital system or health care organization, a personal health record (PHR) is controlled by the patient. Health care facilities and clinical practices are increasing their use of EMRs. In the USA, EMR adoption has been accelerated by federal legislation that enforces clinicians to achieve "meaningful use" with certified EMRs. As a result, physicians are progressively placing more electronic

S.L. Park, M.D. (✉)
Division of Informatics, Department of Pathology,
University of Alabama at Birmingham, Birmingham, AL, USA
e-mail: seungp@uab.edu

A.V. Parwani, M.D., Ph.D., M.B.A. • L. Pantanowitz, M.D.
Department of Pathology, University of Pittsburgh Medical Center,
Pittsburgh, PA, USA
e-mail: parwaniav@upmc.edu; pantanowitzl@upmc.edu

L. Pantanowitz and A.V. Parwani (eds.), *Practical Informatics for Cytopathology*, Essentials in Cytopathology 14, DOI 10.1007/978-1-4614-9581-9_13, © Springer Science+Business Media New York 2014

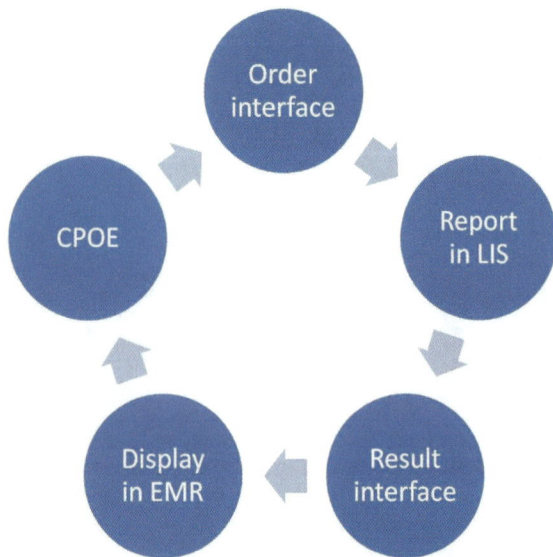

FIG. 13.1 The electronic medical record (EMR)–laboratory information system (LIS) feedback loop. Following computerized provider order entry (CPOE) in the EMR for a lab test, the electronic order gets transmitted via an interface to the LIS. Once the final pathology report gets signed out in the LIS, it is sent in electronic format via another interface into the EMR, where it can be viewed by the ordering clinician. Failure to close this data loop can result in lost orders and/or missing results in the patient's medical record

orders for lab tests in the EMR (Fig. 13.1). They also prefer to look up their patients' results in the EMR. Since this paperless clinical practice is beginning to impact cytology, it is essential for cytopathology laboratories to be aware of this informatics trend.

Pros and Cons

Overall, the benefits of EMR implementation outweigh the problems encountered with this technology. Compared to paper charts, the EMR provides greater portability of information that can be accessed by multiple users. Electronic data is more flexible and therefore can be customized. It is also easier to navigate and search for information, and reduces the need for physical storage space. Data capture is often of better quality and validity than illegible hand written notes. Additional advantages of the EMR include the ability to use decision support tools to standardize care (e.g., restrict test order menus, care sets promote evidence-based medicine), reduce costs (e.g., decrease redundant orders), and help minimize errors. Electronic systems automate coding and billing, allow audit trails to be performed if needed, can support user messaging (e.g., results sent to a provider's inbox), and facilitate data mining (for quality improvement, research or business intelligence). Most benefits are cost-saving and practice-improvement measures that may or may not have a directly measurable return on investment (ROI). Apart from the initial expense and need to train users, it is important to be aware that some complaints about the EMR include workflow disruption (e.g., pop-up alerts), lack of interoperability (e.g., interface problems), the inability to access information when there is a downtime, and privacy concerns related to sharing personal health information. Successful EMR implementation in a hospital system involves careful evaluation of clinical workflow, available resources (e.g., finances, IT support), and organizational culture (e.g., physician buy-in). EMR adoption requires cooperation between the Health IT (HIT) culture and the medical culture. Hence, without hiring qualified informatics staff and engaging the proper clinician champions, EMR implementation projects are likely to fail. It is important to point out that since most studies evaluating the efficacy of EHRs were pursued in large academic environments, the results of these studies may not be valid for small community practices. There is always the danger of vendor lock-in: once an expensive EMR has been selected, implemented, and deployed, it becomes monumentally difficult to migrate to another system.

Computerized Provider Order Entry

Computerized provider order entry (CPOE) enables physicians and other qualified providers to place orders electronically, instead of by paper or telephone. CPOE can be used not only for laboratory tests but also for ordering medications and other tests (e.g., radiology imaging). If the EMR is linked electronically via an interface to the laboratory information system (LIS), CPOE with order communication enables a digital feedback loop in which the orders are entered automatically into the LIS and the results of the order are returned automatically into the originating EHR (Fig. 13.1). CPOE can help reduce turnaround times, reduce errors (e.g., avoid hand written orders), lower cost (e.g., prevent duplicate tests), and utilize clinical decision support systems (e.g., assistance with test selection).

Clinical Decision Support

Clinical Decision Support (CDS) tools are rule-based or artificial intelligence-based systems that attempt to utilize decision-making science techniques to assist users in making better decisions. Common CDS tools are listed in Table 13.1. A simple example is alerting a physician about a drug–drug or drug–allergy interaction at the time of ordering prescriptions. CDS interventions that are presented automatically and fit into the workflow of the clinicians are more likely to be used than those that require the physician to go to a system external to the EMR. CDS that recommends actions for the user to take are more effective than those that simply provide assessments. When implemented properly, CDS are more effective than manual processes for decision support.

Standards

As we become more electronically connected it is important to ensure that disparate information systems, including EMRs, support interoperability. Several standards have

TABLE 13.1 Common clinical decision support techniques

Alerts or warnings

Event-driven reminders

Order sets, care plans, and protocols

Performing calculations

Parameter guidance

Smart documentation forms

Relevant data summaries

Patient monitors and dashboards

Predictive and retrospective analysis

Filtered reference information

---

accordingly been developed to facilitate the exchange of electronic health care information. Health Level 7 (HL7) is the most commonly employed interchange standard that defines how electronic messages are transmitted between EHRs. HL7 provides a set of rules that permits data to be shared and processed by health care organizations in a uniform and consistent manner. Several other standard coding systems that are used to electronically encode data in the EMR are Systematized Nomenclature of Medicine (SNOMED), Current Procedural Terminology (CPT), Logical Observations Identifiers Names and Codes (LOINC), and International Classification of Diseases (ICD). Digital Imaging and Communications in Medicine (DICOM) is the standard used for medical imaging. DICOM is the universal format used to handle images in the radiology Picture Archiving and Communication System (PACS). It should be noted that, despite all these standards, it is often a daunting IT undertaking to get two EHRs to interface with each other, sometimes even when these information systems are provided by the same vendor!

Health Information Exchange

HIE is the transmission of health care information electronically across organizations not only within hospital systems but also across large regions. In the USA, the Health Information Technology for Economic and Clinical Health (HITECH) portion of the American Recovery and Reinvestment Act (ARRA) of 2009 has mandated the nationwide use of EMRs, and also defined success criteria by way of "meaningful use" metrics (Table 13.2). A major challenge facing health care today is that patient medical information often gets trapped in silos of legacy systems,

TABLE 13.2 Meaningful use stages

Stage 1 (2011–2012)	Stage 2 (2014)	Stage 3 (2016)
Electronically capturing health information in a standardized format	More rigorous health information exchange (HIE)	Improving quality, safety, and efficiency, leading to improved health outcomes
Using that information to track key clinical conditions	Increased requirements for e-prescribing and incorporating lab results	Decision support for national high-priority conditions
Communicating that information for care coordinating processes	Electronic transmission of patient care summaries across multiple settings	Patient access to self-management tools
Initiating the reporting of clinical quality measures and public health information	More patient controlled data	Access to comprehensive patient data through patient-centered HIE
Using information to engage patients and their families in their care		Improving population health

unable to be shared. Regional Health Information Organizations (RHIOs) are a group of organizations with a business stake in trying to integrate and exchange health care information with all members of the health care community (hospitals, medical societies, payers, and employers). RHIOs are the building blocks of the proposed National Health Information Network (NHIN).

Chapter 14
Digital Imaging

Milon Amin, Anil V. Parwani, and Liron Pantanowitz

Introduction

We may never have seen Joseph Nicéphore Niépce's "View from the Window at Le Gras" in 1827, were it not for the power of photography as he saw it. He was one of the inventors of photography. Yet, careful processing by the research laboratory of the Eastman Kodak Company was required to most closely represent the image, as seen through Nicéphore's eyes. Well over a century later, the challenge of capturing images "exactly as the observer sees it" remains. Rapid advances in the field of digital pathology have occurred in the last decade, with major impacts on the practice of cytopathology. Each step of the imaging process, which includes image

M. Amin, M.D. (✉)
Affiliated Pathologists Medical Group, Torrance, CA, USA
e-mail: mamin@affiliatedpath.com

A.V. Parwani, M.D., Ph.D., M.B.A. • L. Pantanowitz, M.D.
Department of Pathology, University of Pittsburgh Medical Center, Pittsburgh, PA, USA
e-mail: pantanowitzl@upmc.edu; parwaniav@upmc.edu

L. Pantanowitz and A.V. Parwani (eds.), *Practical Informatics for Cytopathology*, Essentials in Cytopathology 14, DOI 10.1007/978-1-4614-9581-9_14, © Springer Science+Business Media New York 2014

TABLE 14.1 Digital pathology uses

Primary diagnosis
Second opinion (consultation)
Telepathology
Quality assurance
Proficiency testing
Archiving
Education
Image analysis
Research
Marketing
Tracking (audits)

acquisition, storage, manipulation and viewing, may impact the final result, as perceived by the cytologist who views the image. Therefore, it is important that cytologists are familiar with digital imaging technology so that they can harness the power of digital pathology.

There are several uses for digital pathology (Table 14.1). These applications have improved with the evolution from static images to digitization of entire glass slides, also called whole slide imaging (WSI) or virtual microscopy. Digital pathology is an exciting field with continuous disruptive advances in technology, ongoing optimization of pathology workstations, ever-increasing applications for mobile computing, fine-tuning of digital workflow to support a "slide-less" laboratory, and new image analysis tools for better quantification of biomarkers and computer aided diagnosis (CAD), as well as emerging regulatory and legal issues.

Imaging Basics

The fundamental unit in each image is the picture element, also known as the "pixel." In each image, rectangular pixels are arranged in rows and columns (e.g., 1920×1080 pixels).

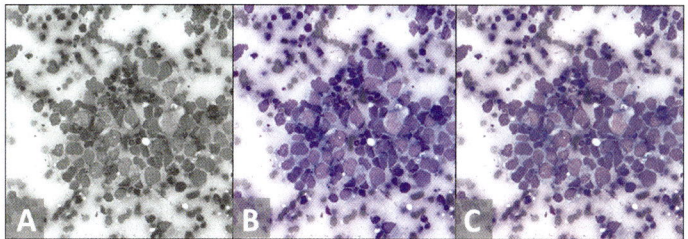

FIG. 14.1 Image modes in Adobe Photoshop. A digital image of small cell carcinoma is shown with (**a**) grayscale, (**b**) RGB color, and (**c**) CMYK color image modes

Alternatively, images can be measured in megapixels, which are the product of the column and row pixel count of the image, divided by 1,000,000 (e.g., 1920 × 1080 pixels is equivalent to 2.0736 megapixels). In addition to pixel resolution, all pixels in an image also have a color value. With the red, blue and green (RGB) model, colors in an image represent a combination of red, blue, and green lights as viewed on a monitor. However, because printed images for publication are produced using various inks (as opposed to colors of light), many publishers recommend that the color model be changed to CMYK (cyan, magenta, yellow, black) so that the printed image matches the digital images as closely as possible (Fig. 14.1). Bit depth refers to the number of color choices per pixel (e.g., An 8-BIT image has 256 colors available).

Image Resolution

The detail of an image is referred to as image resolution—the greater the detail, the higher the resolution. Pixel resolution (measured in pixels) = image width × height. The term "pixels per inch" or ppi is used to describe the resolution of an image to be printed within a specified space. The more pixels there are per inch, the greater the resolution (Fig. 14.2). When the image is displayed on a monitor, image resolution is referred to as "dots per inch" or dpi. For instance, a 100 × 100 pixel

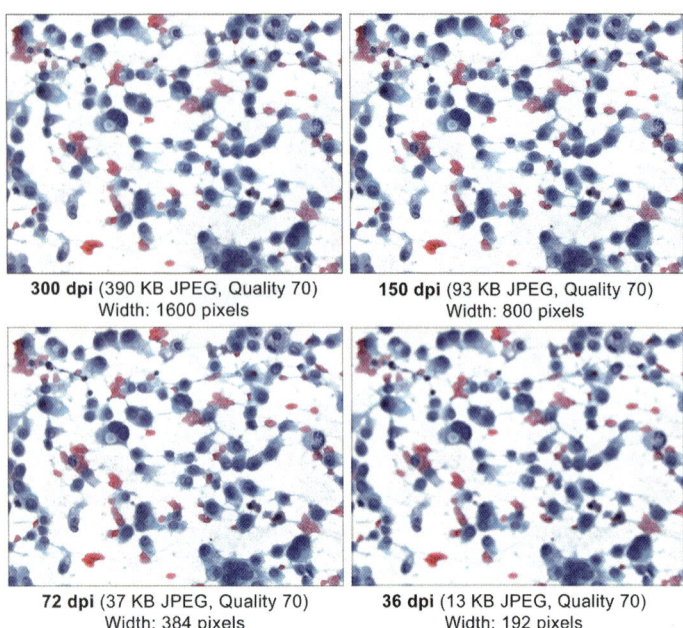

300 dpi (390 KB JPEG, Quality 70)
Width: 1600 pixels

150 dpi (93 KB JPEG, Quality 70)
Width: 800 pixels

72 dpi (37 KB JPEG, Quality 70)
Width: 384 pixels

36 dpi (13 KB JPEG, Quality 70)
Width: 192 pixels

Fɪɢ. 14.2 These figures show the relationship between image resolution (quality) and pixel density. As the pixel density (dpi) decreases so too does the resolution ("quality" of the image)

image printed in a 1-in. square has a resolution of 100 ppi. When examined from a distance of 14 in., the human eye typically cannot resolve individual pixels in an image above 300 ppi. Therefore, 300 ppi is often considered a minimum requirement for publication quality images. However, an assigned ppi value of an image can be misleading. For example, digital images from many cameras are automatically saved with a value of 72 ppi. Furthermore, images opened by image editing programs such as Photoshop may be assigned a default ppi value, irrespective of the resolution of that file. If a program such as Photoshop assigns 72 ppi as a default resolution to an image from a 10 megapixel camera, it is incorrect to say that this image truly has a resolution of

72 ppi, since it is the software program that assigns this value. In such cases, it may be necessary to change the ppi value in the image editing software to 300 or higher, so that the publisher will not mistakenly reject the image.

Digital Cameras

There are several methods to acquire a digital microscopic image in cytology. Digital cameras can be attached to microscopes using a C-mount adapter or to the eyepieces of a light microscope (Fig. 14.3). A telephoto macro lens can, in some cases, substitute for the use of an oil immersion objective lens, because the increased magnification takes place at the eyepiece level rather than the objective lens. Different cameras may be suitable for light microscopy or fluorescent work. Such cameras are connected to desktop computers, which may require the use of a card adapter or dongle (hardware key). Smartphones are becoming increasingly popular to acquire images, especially for telepathology. Light entering a camera lens passes to a sensor, typically called a charge-coupled

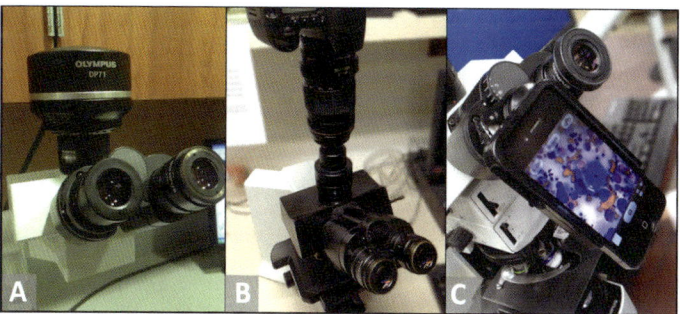

FIG. 14.3 Digital cameras for light microscopy. (**a**) A digital camera head is shown attached to a microscope with a C-mount adapter. (**b**) Digital single lens reflex camera (DSLR) with a 300 mm zoom lens used to capture high magnification images. (**c**) Cell phone with a digital camera mounted to a microscope using a smartphone adapter

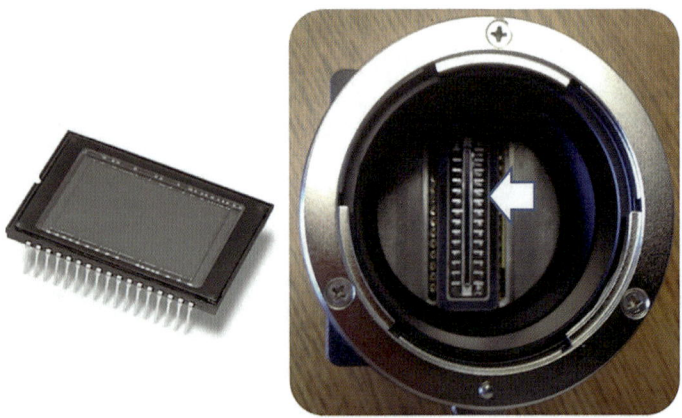

Fig. 14.4 Charge-coupled device (CCD) sensor (*left*). Whole slide scanners that employ line scanning typically have a linear image sensor (*arrow*) in their digital cameras, to permit long image strips to be captured (*right*)

device (CCD) (Fig. 14.4). The CCD converts light into a digital image. The resolution of a digital camera is often limited by this image sensor. With each new generation of cameras comes the ability to obtain higher resolution images (i.e., sensors with more megapixels).

Image File Formats

Images can be saved in a variety of formats (Table 14.2). For static cytology images, the two common formats used are the joint photographic experts group (JPEG) and tagged image file format (TIFF). JPEG involves compression of the images (called lossy compression), resulting in conveniently small image sizes at the expense of image degradation if there is too much compression. TIFF files can be saved without compression (called lossless compression) to retain details, but are typically larger files. Contrary to popular belief, JPEG images with light compression are often indistinguishable to

TABLE 14.2 Select digital image file types

File type (file extension)	Description
Joint photographic experts group (JPG, JPEG)	A standardized file format for photographic image files. Images are subject to degradation if high compression is used. JPEG 2000 offers both lossy and lossless compression with better compression ratios
Tagged image file format (TIF, TIFF)	A common file format that supports a variety of color models, compression options, or uncompressed formats to preserve image quality
Bitmap (BMP)	An uncompressed file type that, although widely supported, is not commonly used in presentation or publication formats
Photoshop document (PSD)	An uncompressed file type accessible only through image editing formats such as Adobe Photoshop
Digital imaging and communications in medicine (DICOM)	A standardized file format used in medicine, predominately in radiology, with embedded metadata for patient identification

the naked eye from TIFF images (Fig. 14.5) JPEG images are therefore useful in presentations and even for telecytology, particularly if the transmission of large files is of concern. Digitized slides (whole slide images) are large files (sometimes several GB in size). Moreover, because different WSI scanners may save their files in proprietary formats (e.g., .svs for Aperio, .ngr for Hamamatsu, .scn for Leica., .vsi for Olympus, and .mrxs for 3D-Histech), these images cannot be easily shared and viewed using other WSI systems. OpenSlide (available at http://openslide.org/) provides a simple interface to read several different whole slide images. Digital Imaging and Communications in Medicine (DICOM) is the standard for handling medical (mainly radiology) images. DICOM supplements 122 and 145 for pathology have been created to promote interoperability using whole slide images.

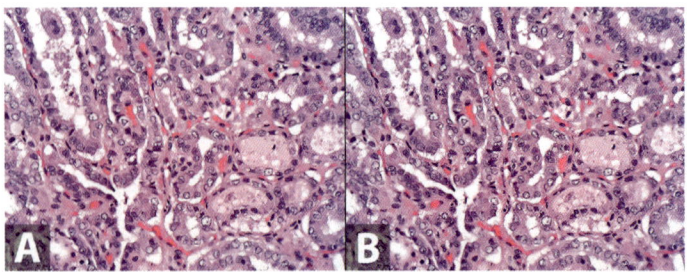

Fig. 14.5 Comparison of a (**a**) TIFF image (5.4 MB) and a (**b**) lightly compressed JPEG image (0.9 MB, Quality 70). In print on this page, these images are essentially indistinguishable to the naked eye

Post-processing Optimization

The quality of a digital image depends on more than just focus and resolution. There are several other parameters such as white balance, color levels, and saturation that also play an important role in image quality. While some of these factors can be adjusted at the time of image acquisition, post-processing using software such as Adobe Photoshop, or the free alternative GIMP (GNU Image Manipulation Program), can be used to enhance images. A common scenario with podium presentations is where the speaker's images appear blurry in PowerPoint or Keynote, even if high resolution images were originally obtained. This occurs because the images get downsized to match the resolution of the screen. For example, a 5 megapixel (2560×1920) image can get downsized to the projector's EXtended Graphics Array (XGA) resolution (1024×768). Sharpening an image (i.e., making it appear more "crisp") may partly compensate for this effect. While sharpening options are available in PowerPoint, they are not as robust and precise as those used in dedicated image processing software. A proposed alternative technique is to resize the image to the resolution of the projector that will be used for the presentation (currently 1024×768 at most national meetings) (Fig. 14.6).

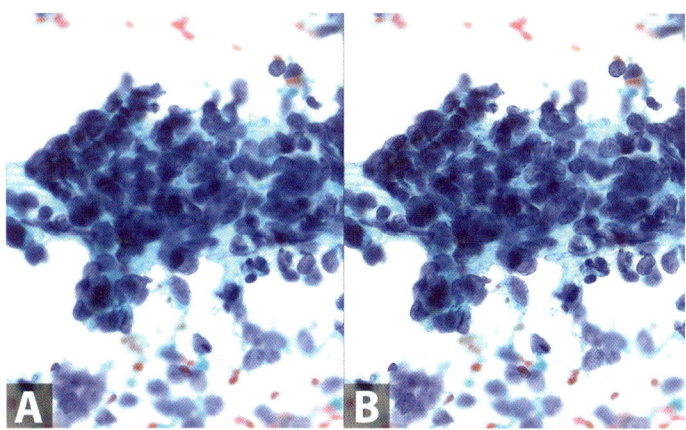

FIG. 14.6 Comparison of images viewed in Microsoft PowerPoint. (**a**) TIFF image at 1600×1200. (**b**) JPEG image at 1024×768 with sharpening. Note the increased "sharpness" in the JPEG image, despite the lower resolution and compressed format

White Balance

White balance is the process that makes white objects or backgrounds appear white in a digital image. The reason to adjust white balance is to get all of the colors in an image as accurate as possible. White balance can be performed before an image is taken using the camera's settings, or afterwards using image-editing software (Fig. 14.7). Using these tools to select an area of the image that should be white not only corrects the background color to white, but will also adjust the surrounding elements to match as well.

Color Adjustment

Setting the white balance alone may not resolve the full gamut of perceived color in an image. Sometimes basophilic areas may appear more "blue" than violet, and eosinophilic areas more "red" than pink or magenta. Image-editing

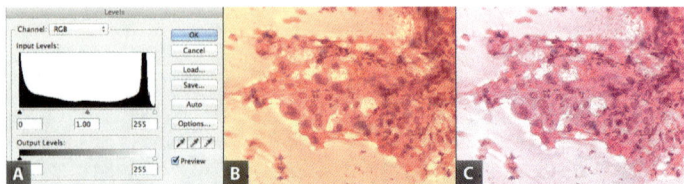

FIG. 14.7 Impact of manual white balance performed post-processing. (**a**) Histogram in image-editing software showing the white balance tool. The histogram summarizes the distribution of "light" and "dark" areas within the image. (**b**) Original image without adjusted white balance; note the *yellow* cast (tint). (**c**) Image after applying white balance

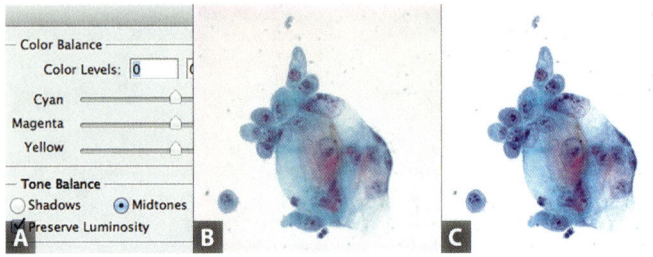

FIG. 14.8 Use of the "color balance" tool in Adobe Photoshop. (**a**) Color balance options window. (**b**) Original image. (**c**) Enhanced image after increasing the "*red*" and "*blue*" parameters in the midtones

software tools such as "color balance" and "selective color" allow one to manually adjust for these differences without affecting other colors of the image (Fig. 14.8). While software suites include options for "auto color" and "auto levels," applying these tools may not necessarily yield desirable results with cytology images (Fig. 14.9).

Sharpening

Perceiving an image as "sharp" involves interpretation of resolution and acutance (contrast). Resolution refers to the recorded detail by a lens/sensor combination. Acutance

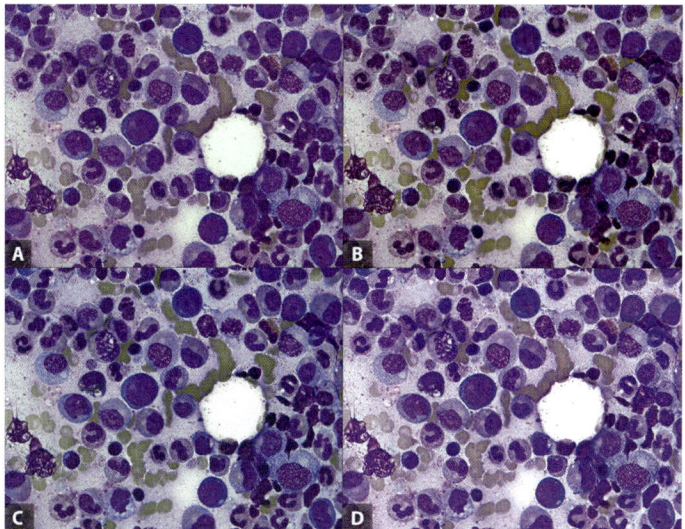

Fig. 14.9 Impact of "automatic" color and level adjustments of a digital image. (**a**) Original image. (**b**) Image after "auto-color" adjustment in Adobe Photoshop. (**c**) Image after "auto-levels" adjustment in Adobe Photoshop. Note the distorted "*green*" color of the erythrocytes after these adjustments. (**d**) Image after only applying white balance

refers to the lowest tone difference a lens/sensor combination can record. Most lens/sensor combinations have high resolution, but low acutance; they can capture abundant detail, but such detail may not always be apparent. This "hidden" detail can be enhanced by using sharpening tools (i.e., correct a "blurred" image). However, misuse of sharpening tools can lead to artifacts in images such as halos, aliasing ("jagged edges"), and noise.

Imaging Process and Management

The digital imaging process involves four steps (capture–save–edit–share) (Fig. 14.10). Saving digital images, especially many images of large file size, requires a robust and scalable

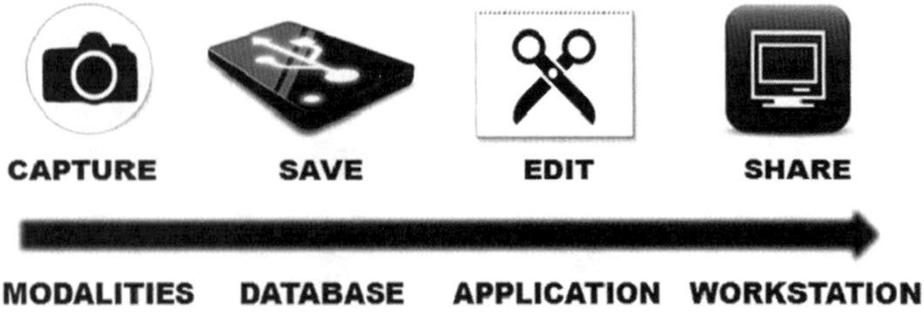

CAPTURE   SAVE   EDIT   SHARE

MODALITIES   DATABASE   APPLICATION   WORKSTATION

Fig. 14.10 Steps involved in the digital imaging process. Step 1 involves image capture (acquisition) using various devices (e.g., digital camera, WSI scanner). Step 2 involves saving the image file (archiving) in an organized fashion (e.g., to a database). Step 3 involves potential editing (e.g., annotation, cropping) of the image using specific application software. Step 4 involves sharing (e.g., transmitting) an image to be viewed on a computer monitor (workstation)

file storage platform. Cost may be a significant impediment for retaining all images. Digital images in pathology can either be integrated directly into the laboratory information system (LIS) or be housed in a separate (modular) system. If images are saved directly into the LIS, metadata (e.g., case number) accompanying the image is also automatically stored in the LIS database. Although images saved in a separate repository may not be automatically linked to corresponding cases in the LIS at the time they are acquired, they can still be imported into the LIS. The major advantage of the latter approach is that it provides greater flexibility (e.g., many more imaging modalities can be supported, and it is often easier to manipulate and share images). Commercial middleware is available to help users automatically feed images into their LIS. The contemporary LIS is beginning to resemble the Picture Archiving and Communication System (PACS) used in radiology to store, distribute, and display their images.

Whole Slide Imaging

A limitation of conventional photomicrography is the inability to provide sufficient and focused digital images that represent the entire slide. WSI attempts to solve this problem by

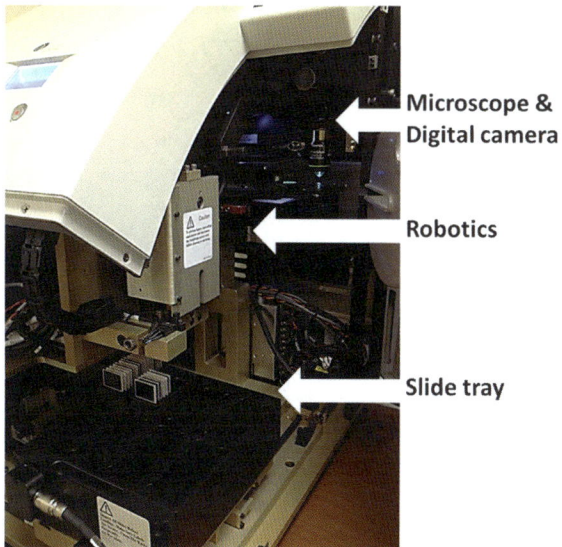

Fig. 14.11 Whole slide scanner hardware components

scanning (digitizing) the entire glass slide at high resolution. The instrument used for this purpose produces many images that get "stitched together" to generate a large image. Such whole slide images may exceed 40,000 pixels in length and 4 gigabytes (GB) in size. The quality of the images produced is generally of diagnostic quality, and simulates viewing the slide with a conventional microscope (i.e., virtual microscopy). Most published validation studies indicate that with user training, WSI platforms can be used to make diagnoses that are as accurate as those made by light microscopy. The components of a WSI scanner include a slide tray (loader), robotics, optical microscope, digital camera, computer hardware and software (for image scanning, compression, management, and viewing) (Fig. 14.11). The footprint of WSI scanners varies, and includes devices that may allow just 1–2 slides to be scanned to those that can accommodate hundreds of slides to be automatically scanned (Fig. 14.12). Newer WSI scanners also have the ability for users to remotely control the microscope for telepathology.

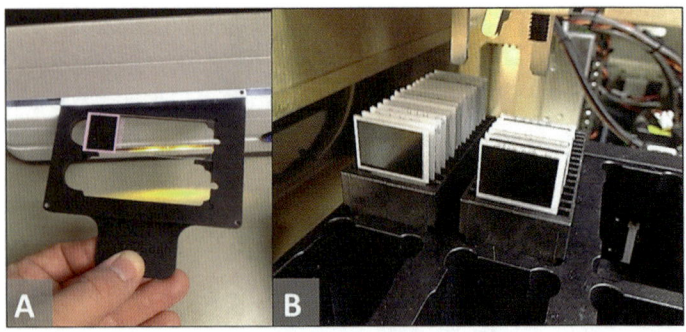

Fig. 14.12 Whole slide scanner (**a**) that allows only a few slides to be uploaded at once and (**b**) one that can automatically scan many slides

Glass slides can be digitized at multiple magnifications (e.g., 20×, 40×). For scanning routine surgical pathology H and E slides, 20× is often adequate. However, cytology slides should ideally be scanned at 40×. Unfortunately, this takes longer to perform and also generates larger digital files. A slide can also be scanned in multiple focal planes (X, Y, and Z axes) (Fig. 14.13). A particular problem in cytology is that many scanners only capture one level of the Z-axis (i.e., depth of focus) for the entire scanned area. This poses a problem for those cytology cases that have thick smears or three-dimensional cell clusters, where the pathologist must "focus up and down" to see everything clearly. More recent scanners have the capability of performing Z-stacking (i.e., capturing multiple levels of the Z-axis).

Viewing Whole-Slide Images

Most digital slide viewers used to view and navigate a digital slide are proprietary. As noted above, OpenSlide is a C library that provides an interface to read several whole slide images. Using viewer software, cytologists can pan around an image and zoom in to examine virtual slides at different

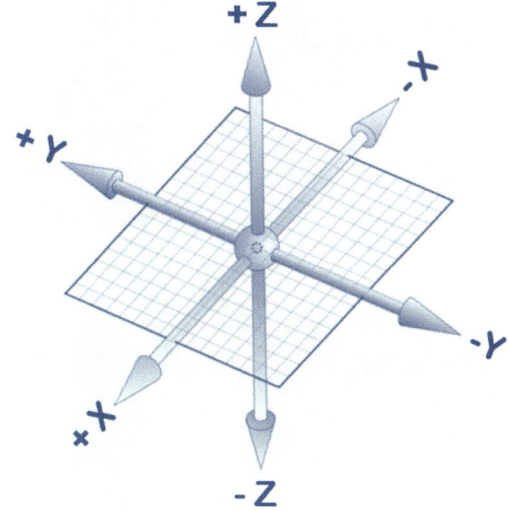

Fɪɢ. 14.13 *X*, *Y*, and *Z* axes. Scanning a slide along the *X* and *Y* *horizontal* axes allows the user to pan around the entire slide. Scanning the slide along the *Z* axis (*vertical*) allows the user to see the different focal planes of the scanned image

magnifications. Screening of digital cytology slides can be facilitated by exploiting certain software features such as auto panning, tracking and simultaneous slide review. Viewers also offer tools to annotate (e.g., mark or measure areas) images (Fig. 14.14). Some software may also permit teleconferencing, allowing multiple remote users to simultaneously log in and view the same image (e.g., for teleconsultation).

Image Displays

Digital images can be viewed using various displays ranging from medical grade to commercial computer monitors, as well as tablets (e.g., iPad) and smartphones. The most common type of display used is the liquid crystal display (LCD). Several parameters in these displays such as monitor size

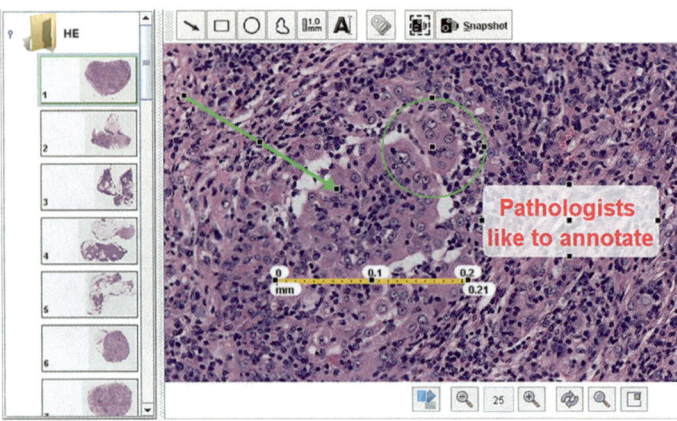

FIG. 14.14 Annotated whole slide image using viewer software tools

(measured diagonally in inches), display resolution, aspect ratio, refresh rate, luminance, power consumption, and so on can affect the quality of an image. For clinical practice, the diagnostic digital "cockpit" where a cytologist is expected to view and interpret digital images also needs to provide access to other required data (e.g., lab information system, electronic medical record, online resources).

Image Analysis

One of the major advantages of digital images is the ability to employ image analysis tools for CAD. Manual methods based on human visual inspection for counting (e.g., Ki67 index) or to provide a semiquantitative score of an immunostain (e.g., HER2/neu 0, 1+, 2+, and 3+) are subject to inter-laboratory and interobserver variability. Manual methods are also imprecise and of low sensitivity. Image analysis using software algorithms allows these tasks to be automated. Computer-assisted analysis is also more accurate and reproducible. In general, image analysis is a multistep process that involves feature extraction, feature selection, dimensionality reduction, and classification steps. Image analysis can be used to identify rare events, provide quantitative measurements, and/or recognize spatial patterns of specific features.

Multispectral Imaging

Microscopy using multispectral imaging refers to the capture of spectrally resolved information (colors at different wavelengths) at each pixel in an image. Spectral microscopy can use bright field and/or fluorescence. This technique allows tissues to be analyzed that have been simultaneously labeled with multiple immunostains. Multiplexing many antibody labels is a desirable way to conservatively discover new biomarkers with small tissue samples.

Chapter 15
Automated Pap Tests

Liron Pantanowitz

Introduction

A decade ago very few cytology laboratories were engaged in automated cytology. Since then, several automated preparation devices have been introduced including instruments for cell collection from liquid samples, monolayer slide preparation, and autostainers. Computers were interfaced with cytology microscope stages (e.g., AcCell Series 2000, Pathfinder System, Cytosafe System) to assist with screening, by ensuring that all fields on a slide were examined. Manual Pap test screening remained a challenge because this task was (and still is) repetitive, labor-intensive, suffers from a significant false negative rate, carries ergonomic risk, and can be affected by the screening environment. This difficulty is compounded by the shortage of skilled cytotechnologists, which ushered in the need for automated screening of Pap tests. Early semi-automated screening devices were plagued by lack of a

L. Pantanowitz, M.D. (✉)
Department of Pathology, University of Pittsburgh Medical Center,
Pittsburgh, PA, USA
e-mail: pantanowtizl@upmc.edu

L. Pantanowitz and A.V. Parwani (eds.), *Practical Informatics for Cytopathology*, Essentials in Cytopathology 14, DOI 10.1007/978-1-4614-9581-9_15,
© Springer Science+Business Media New York 2014

147

standardized sample, the conventional Pap smear, that was conducive to rapid digital image acquisition and computer processing. This resulted in the advent of Liquid-Based Cytology (LBC) with production of a cellular "monolayer" on a glass slide. Today, advances in computing, innovative software and digital imaging technology have been leveraged to successfully automate Pap test screening.

In order to accomplish this task, conventional Pap smears were converted to liquid-based samples from which a monolayer of cells on a slide could be prepared and stained using standardized staining protocols. LBC solved two main problems, viz., (1) pre-analytic issues because now sampling, fixation, staining, obscuring background material and artifacts (e.g., overlapping cells) were improved and variables in slide quality were now under the control of the cytology laboratory; and (2) analytic problems because the cell spots presented a smaller area on a slide to screen/image and monolayers in general were easier to read. Today, two different LBC Pap tests are available including ThinPrep and SurePath methods (Table 15.1). MonoPrep is no longer available. An additional advantage of LBC is that residual vial material can be utilized to make additional slides and/or perform other diagnostic tests (e.g., HPV, microbiology and molecular testing, cell block, immunocytochemistry).

Both primary and interactive automated screening systems are available (Fig. 15.1). The only primary screening device available is the FocalPoint Slide Profiler. Such primary screening systems classify slides as requiring cytotechnologist review versus no review, as well as provide additional information associated with likelihood of abnormality. Interactive systems guide cytotechnologists to targeted areas of cells on a slide for their review. The cells are scanned using algorithms that analyze many (e.g., over 400) cellular characteristics. Imaging algorithms are designed to detect specimen adequacy (according to The Bethesda System slide adequacy criteria), benign cellular changes, infections, and morphologic changes associated with epithelial abnormalities. The location of these cells is recorded, which is used to provide relocation coordinates on the glass slide for visual review.

TABLE 15.1 Computer-assisted screening timeline

Date	Event (US only)
1923	Pap test introduced by Dr. Papanicolaou, but only commonly used after late 1940s
1925	PAPNET system is FDA approved for rescreening
1996	ThinPrep Pap test is FDA approved
1998	BD FocalPoint Slide Profiler (AutoPap 300 QC) is FDA approved for primary screening
1999	Autocyte Prep (now BD SurePath) Pap test is FDA approved
2001	BD FocalPoint Slide Profiler is approved to screen SurePath slides
2002	ThinPrep Imaging System is FDA approved
2006	MonoPrep Pap test is introduced
2008	BD FocalPoint GS Imaging System is FDA approved (in the USA for SurePath only)

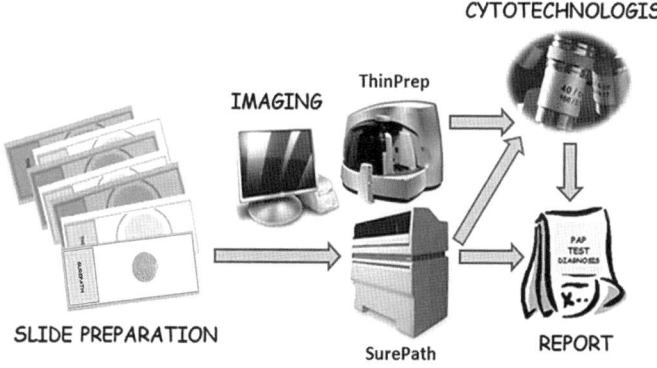

CYTOTECHNOLOGIST

IMAGING ThinPrep

SLIDE PREPARATION SurePath REPORT

FIG. 15.1 Automated Pap test screening workflow using different imaging systems. Properly prepared glass slides are loaded onto imaging devices to be screened. ThinPrep slides get reviewed by a cytotechnologist before a report gets issued. With SurePath slides imaged on the BD FocalPoint Slide Profiler the laboratory has the option to use the "No Further Review" feature, which allows for up to 25 % of the slides most likely to be negative based on ranking to be reported out without cytotech review. The remaining 75 % of SurePath slides undergo full slide review (including negative and abnormal cases). (Image adapted from Khalbuss et al. Quick Compendium of Cytopathology. Chicago: ASCP Press; 2013)

Performance of automated screening systems has been positive. Reported benefits include increased sensitivity of abnormal Pap test diagnoses including squamous intraepithelial lesion (SIL) detection, fewer false negative cases and increased productivity. This technology also resulted in increased pathologist-referred cases. Limitations include an initial user "learning curve," increase in ASCUS rates, as well as equipment and maintenance costs. Automated Pap test screening has been shown to be cost-effective in high volume cytology laboratories. In a minority of cases, computer-assisted imaging devices may fail to detect atypical/neoplastic glandular cells of interest within selected fields of view (FOV). The CLIA regulated maximum of 200 LBC Paps per screening day for a cytotechnologist is now recognized as unrealistic and dangerous. Changes to Federal Regulations are being considered.

Technology

Imaging systems employ a combination of microscopes, digital/video cameras, and computers to accomplish automated screening. LBC processed and stained glass slides get loaded in batches in slide cassettes or onto slide trays which then get placed into an imaging instrument (referred to as an imaging station or slide profiler). This imaging equipment is linked to a computer (sometimes called an image processor controller) (Fig. 15.2). The accession identification (ID) number on the slide gets read using an optical character recognition camera. The slide label must have the correct accession ID to be scanned and it needs to be correctly positioned on the slide in order for the reader to locate it. The area with cellular material on the slide (cell spot) is then automatically scanned (imaged) and analyzed. Fiducial marks on ThinPrep slides are used to guide slide scanning. It takes about 4–6 min to process each slide. Imaging may be impaired by slides with wet media, bubbles, dirt and fingerprints, or if they are incorrectly labeled or loaded. The device may also be

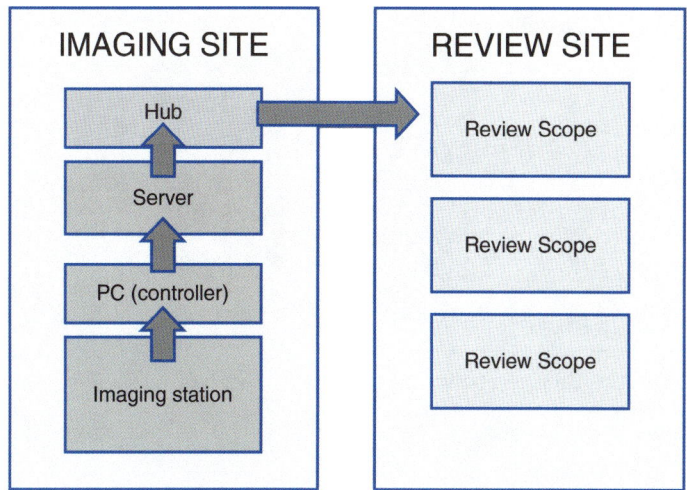

FIG. 15.2 Schematic of the network for a Pap test imaging system

sensitive to vibrations. Slides with coverslips that extend beyond the slide edge or labels with lifted edges may cause slides to get broken and/or damage the instrument. Data including the slide ID and various image-related data (e.g., coordinates or reference frames for imaged objects of interest, ranking of cellular abnormality, cell pattern images, specimen quality indicators) for select FOVs are stored on a nearby networked server (data manager) within a centralized database.

System database queries can be performed and reports can be generated if needed (e.g., logs, usage history, slide data records, workload summary, and errors). Coordinates are saved for future relocation. A review station/scope which communicates with the server is used by the cytotechnologist to subsequently review imaged slides (Figs. 15.3 and 15.4). Review scopes/stations can be located away (e.g., 100 m) from the server. For further distances additional network hubs will be needed. For facilities where slide imaging and

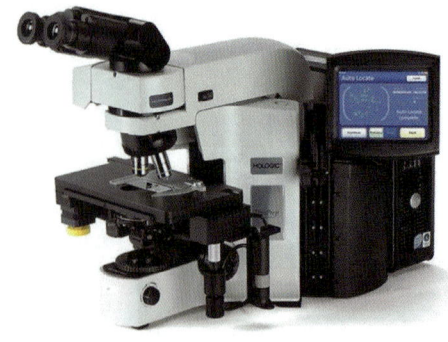

FIG. 15.3 ThinPrep review scope (courtesy of HOLOGIC, Inc. and affiliates)

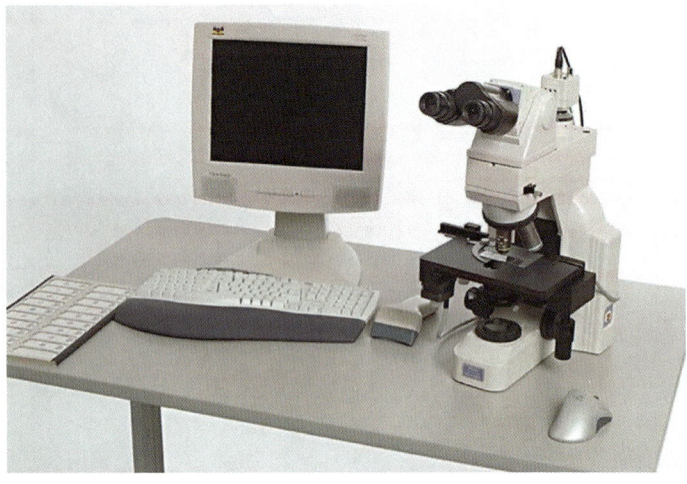

FIG. 15.4 BD FocalPoint review station (courtesy of BD Diagnostics)

cytotechnologist review of slides are remotely located, slide data may need to be exported (e.g., on to CD ROM) from the imaging site and shipped with the patient slides to the remote review site. Review scopes/stations have microscopes with stages set-up to relocate the FOV using X and Y

coordinates. Scanning the glass slide's ID number at the review scope/station retrieves data (FOV coordinates) from the server. Scopes may permit cells of interest within a target zone to be electronically marked by the cytotechnologist. Newer review scopes have a smaller footprint and therefore take up less space. They are also better ergonomically designed including touch screen user-friendly screen interfaces.

Primary Screening Systems

These computer-assisted screening systems perform primary screening without cytotechnologist interaction. Technology currently used in this manner is the BD FocalPoint Slide Profiler (BD Diagnostics-TriPath), formerly known as the AutoPap System. This system was FDA approved for both conventional smears and BD SurePath Pap tests. Using this system, glass slides are scanned, during which a computer assigns scores using population-based statistical analysis tools. Each slide is scanned in total and then assigned a ranking score (0–1). The closer the score is to 1, the more likely the slide is to be abnormal. The ranking is done in relation to other slides that were scanned in the group. Ranking information is further represented by dividing the group of slides into Quintiles. Quintile 1 corresponds to those slides receiving the highest scores. In addition, these systems can identify the highest scoring areas on each slide and provide up to 10 FOVs for guided screening. These systems can also identify a proportion of cases (e.g., up to 15 % of the highest ranking negative slides) for directed quality control (QC) rescreen.

Interactive Screening Systems

These computer-assisted screening devices require a cytotechnologist to interact with the imaging system at a microscope review station in order to interpret Pap tests. Both the ThinPrep Imaging System (Hologic) (Fig. 15.5) and BD

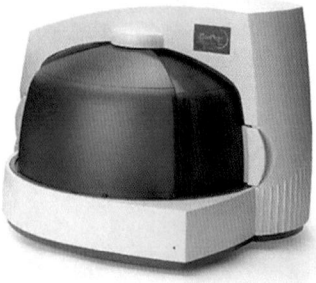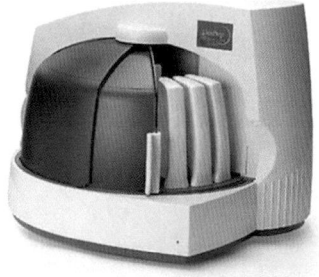

Fig. 15.5 ThinPrep Imaging station. The instrument on the *right* has the sliding door open showing the slide cassettes (courtesy of HOLOGIC, Inc. and affiliates)

FocalPoint GS (Guided Screening) Imaging System (BD Diagnostics—TriPath) are marketed for this purpose. The cytotechnologist's attention is driven to significant cellular fields of interest using automated X–Y axis relocation. The final interpretation relies on the diagnostic acumen of the human reviewer.

Implementation and Maintenance

A new installation may be disruptive for a laboratory when an imager first gets inserted into the workflow. The laboratory is required to validate and document that their new instrument functions as clinically intended and is consistent with the manufacturer's recommendations. Since a proprietary Pap stain will need to be adopted with ThinPrep LBC, cytologists should be aware that this may cause darker nuclear staining of cells. For FocalPoint users the laboratory can use their current Pap stain. Cytologists should also note that their determination of specimen adequacy and diagnosis of infections may be limited to the FOVs selected. Moreover, selected abnormal fields may not necessarily be the most diagnostic. Training staff, instrument calibration and regular maintenance of equipment are important responsibilities of the lab. Instrument service records need to be saved. The operation of these devices should comply with the manufacturer standards. For example, with ThinPrep imaging devices there is a verification slide stored inside the imaging device that should be kept clean; it is used by the imaging system for periodic instrument verification. Data on the server should be regularly exported and backed up. Also, security of the system should be enabled to restrict access to archival data. In the event of instrument failure or downtime the lab needs a policy documenting how they will handle processing slides trapped within the failed device, as well as the alternative procedure (e.g., manual screening) to be used. Once cytotechnologists overcome their initial learning curve with this technology, their productivity can be expected to be increased. Therefore, it is important that cytotechnologist performance is carefully monitored so that they do not exceed maximum workload limits (slides screened/hour). The lab should have a documented workload policy and evidence of data recording for automated screening of cytology slides. Finally, reimbursement (billing) will need to be accordingly adjusted, as specific CPT codes exist for both technical and professional components for imaged Pap tests.

Chapter 16
Telecytology

Sara E. Monaco and Liron Pantanowitz

Introduction

Telecytology involves the remote transmission of cytology images for evaluation at a distance. This technology can be utilized for a variety of reasons including diagnosis, consultation, education, and research (Table 16.1). Apart from the shortage of cytopathologists, with recent advances in digital imaging and networking technology there has been a growing interest in applying telepathology tools in cytopathology. Early publications on telecytology focused on its applications in gynecological cytology. Since then, telecytology has also been employed in non-gynecological cytology, including rapid on-site evaluations of FNA.

For consultations, telecytology can help to obtain an expert opinion (teleconsultation) on a case remotely.

S.E. Monaco, M.D. (✉) • L. Pantanowitz, M.D.
Department of Pathology, University of Pittsburgh Medical Center, Pittsburgh, PA, USA
e-mail: monacose@upmc.edu; pantanowitzl@upmc.edu

L. Pantanowitz and A.V. Parwani (eds.), *Practical Informatics for Cytopathology*, Essentials in Cytopathology 14, DOI 10.1007/978-1-4614-9581-9_16, © Springer Science+Business Media New York 2014

TABLE 16.1 Applications of telecytology

Primary diagnosis
Rapid on-site evaluation
Intraoperative consultation (e.g., brain smears)
Consultation (second opinion)
Education (teleconferences)
Quality assurance (case review)
Examination and assessment (e.g., proficiency testing)

Telecytology thereby provides easy access to experts and in doing so improves patient care. When glass slides are mailed for consultation via the postal system, there is a potential for these slides to get lost or broken. With telecytology this can be avoided since the original slides are retained at the home institution. This is particularly important in cytopathology because cytology slides are often unique and irreplaceable, as opposed to histology tissue blocks from which recuts can be obtained. In addition, tele-consultation may be obtained quicker. For immediate assessments of FNA, pathologists and cytotechnologists are usually required to travel far distances in order to reach the sites where the biopsy is being obtained in order to provide feedback to the performer of the biopsy about specimen adequacy, render a preliminary diagnosis, and appropriately triage the specimen. However, this service utilizes a great deal of time and cytopathologists may not always be readily available. Telecytology offers the ability to view these slides remotely via the electronic transmission of images, which allows the pathologist to stay in his/her office without wasting time traveling and minimizes disruption of their work (Fig. 16.1). The use of telecytology allows for outreach or expansion of cytology services, which may be advantageous in areas that do not have adequate access to cytopathologists.

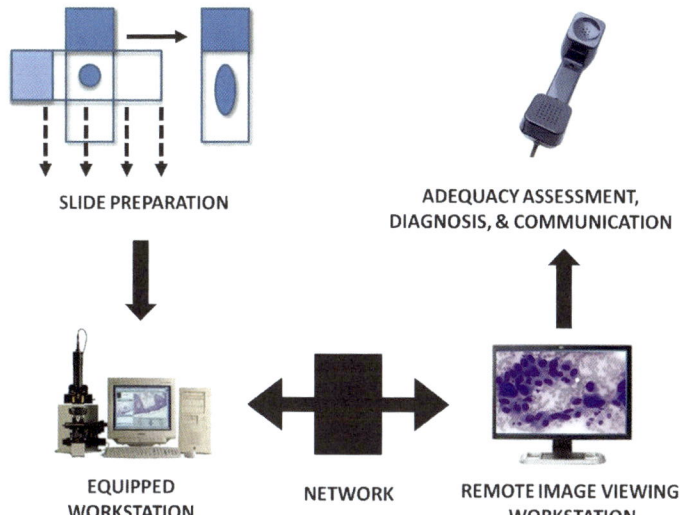

SLIDE PREPARATION

ADEQUACY ASSESSMENT,
DIAGNOSIS, & COMMUNICATION

EQUIPPED
WORKSTATION

NETWORK

REMOTE IMAGE VIEWING
WORKSTATION

Fig. 16.1 Telecytology for rapid on-site evaluation (ROSE). A remote operator (e.g., cytotechnologist, cytology fellow or resident) prepares glass slides, loads these on to an appropriate workstation (e.g., robotic microscope), and transmits images (or video) via a network connection for remote viewing. The remote consulting cytopathologist can communicate with the operator and/or clinician performing the procedure via the telephone

Telecytology Systems

The electronic transmission of cytology images in telecytology can be achieved using static (store and forward), dynamic (real-time), and/or hybrid systems. Three types of devices are used to acquire microscopic digital images, including microscope-mounted cameras, remotely controlled robotic microscopes, and whole slide imaging (WSI) scanners. Microscope-mounted cameras are widely available and can be used to acquire static digital images or stream live video/digital images for remote viewing. Newer WSI scanners have the capability of viewing digitized (static) slides and offering remote control of live images with built-in robotic microscopes.

Static Telecytology

Static (snapshot) digital images obtained with a microscope-mounted camera can be sent by e-mail or saved to a shared server for someone to access and view. The advantage of using static images is that these systems are generally cheaper, easy to implement and maintain, and readily available. Digital files are generally small and manageable (e.g., a few megabytes). Sophisticated software is often not required, as most people have access to e-mail. However, this manual method is labor intensive and requires that the person taking these images is knowledgeable about cytology and what to photograph. Moreover, the images obtained by these cameras can only capture a small field of view (FOV) of the glass slide. Hence, the interpreter has to rely on others for representative image selection (Fig. 16.2). Another disadvantage of static images is the inability to provide dynamic focus (Fig. 16.3).

Live Streaming

Many cytology laboratories rely on remote live telemicroscopy. This can be achieved by using a microscope-mounted video or digital camera. The image obtained with a mounted camera by a person driving the glass slide can be viewed by a cytopathologist remotely either by streaming (continuous transmission) the image in real-time or allowing the pathologist to gain access to the computer workstation (i.e., desktop sharing) that is attached to the microscope in use. This means of telecytology is an affordable option for many labs, is easy to implement, and allows for focusing. However, similar to still images, the quality of interpretation is dependent on the experience and skill of the person who is navigating the slide at the remote site. In addition, the host and consultant will need to be able to communicate in real-time via telephone, online video calling, or with mobile chat (Fig. 16.4).

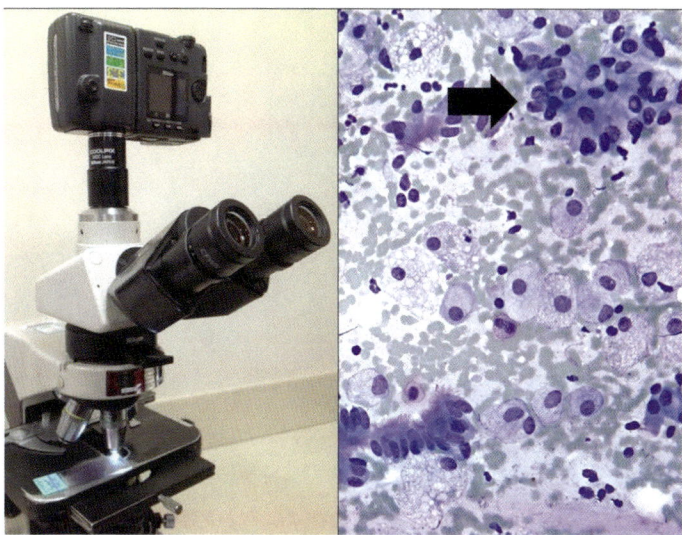

FIG. 16.2 Store and forward telecytology. Typical microscope-mounted camera used to acquire static digital images (*left*). This example illustrates one of the limitations of static telecytology, whereby the wrong field of view (FOV) could be selected by an inexperienced operator, leading to an incorrect diagnosis (*right*). In this image of a lung FNA there are benign ciliated bronchial cells and macrophages, as well as a focus of mucinous adenocarcinoma (*arrow*) that would be important to photograph (FNA aspirate smear, Diff Quik stain, original magnification 400×)

Robotic Telemicroscopy

Remote robotic microscopy offers real-time (or dynamic) simulated examination of the entire glass slide. Pathologists are able to remotely control a robotic microscope stage (for navigation) and objectives (for magnification and focusing) using software installed on their own computer (Fig. 16.5). Robotic telepathology has been used most successfully with intraoperative consultations (e.g., frozen sections). Both the host and recipient require integrated software (Fig. 16.6). Viewing images is relatively slow (e.g., 10 min to view a single slide), and the technology may succumb to

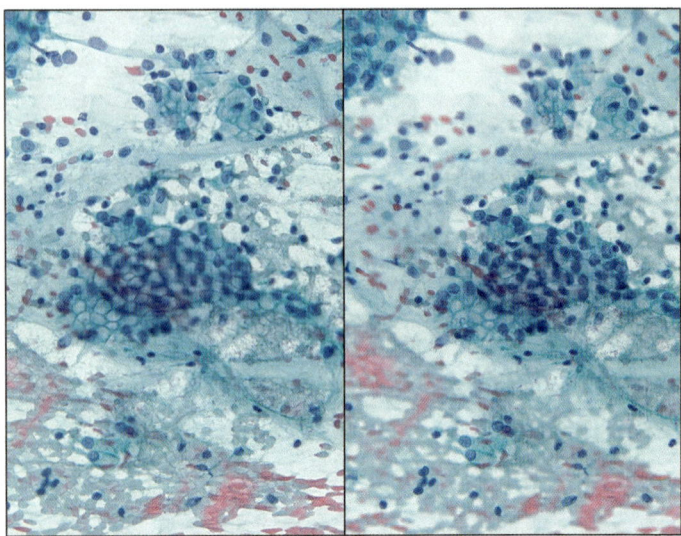

FIG. 16.3 This example illustrates the importance of fine focus when viewing cytology material via static telecytology. The *left* and *right* images show the same field of view (FOV) at different levels of fine focus. Nuclear details of the cell cluster in the center are more clearly defined in the right-sided image (FNA aspirate smear, Papanicolaou stain, original magnification 400×). This is due to the fact that the aspirate smear contains the entire cell on the slide, not just a small slice of the cell, as seen in histological sections

delays in transmission of instructions to the robotic controls. In addition, the equipment is expensive, is difficult to maintain, and has limited use outside of immediate assessments and consultations.

Whole Slide Imaging (Virtual Microscopy)

WSI allows an entire glass slide to be rapidly digitized (automated or manual), archived, and then accessed for viewing. This digitized slide (virtual image) can be visualized on a computer monitor without the use of a microscope, and

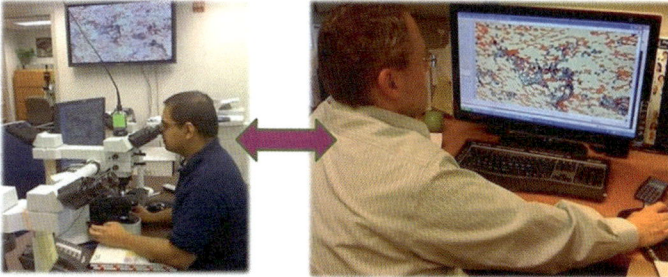

Fellow streaming slides through NetCam package

Cytopathologist reviewing the same slide on his desktop screen

FIG. 16.4 This example illustrates Web-based streaming for an FNA. In order for the host (fellow on the *left* in this example) to transmit an image in real-time to be remotely viewed by the consultant (cytopathologist on the *right* in this example), both individuals need to be able to communicate with each other in real-time and use compatible software

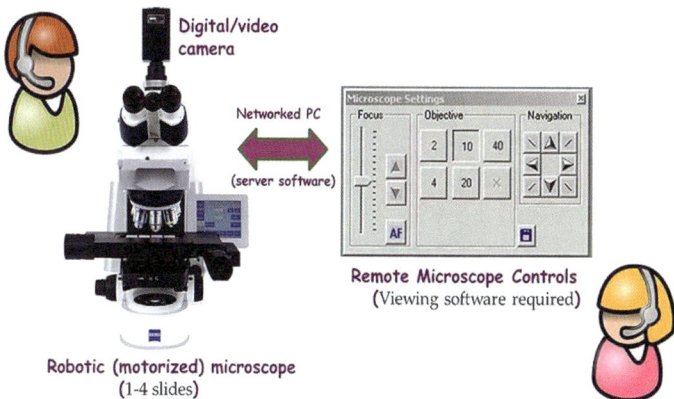

Digital/video camera

Networked PC

(server software)

Remote Microscope Controls
(Viewing software required)

Robotic (motorized) microscope
(1-4 slides)

FIG. 16.5 Schematic of a robotic telecytology system. A host individual (*left*) is required to load glass slides onto a robotic microscope. A cytopathologist (*right*) in communication with the host is able to remotely control this robotic microscope (e.g., focus, objectives, and navigation) using dedicated software from their own computer

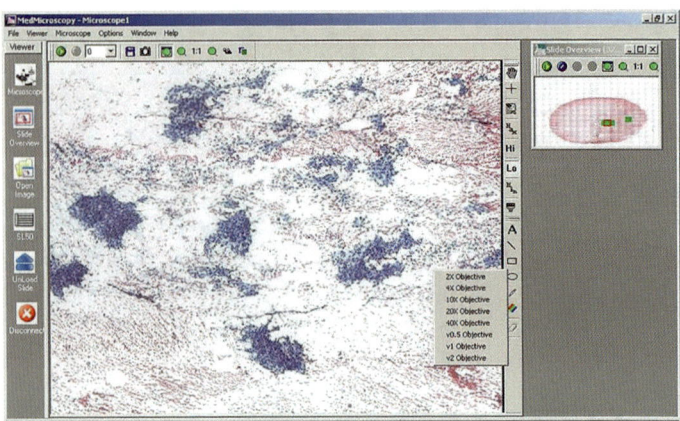

Fɪɢ. 16.6 Screenshot of a digital image being remotely viewed using the image viewer of a robotic telecytology system. Note the small thumbnail image provided in the *upper right* that offers an overview of the entire glass slide. Many icons are available for the user (e.g., to annotate images). (Image courtesy of Dr. Anil Parwani)

permits transmission to one or several remote users simultaneously. WSI is discussed in greater detail in Chap. 15 (digital imaging). This technology allows the entire slide to be available for review and manipulation by a remote user, minimizing the need for an experienced on-site operator for field selection. WSI also produces digital images with high resolution (image quality) that facilitates rapid viewing and has demonstrated high diagnostic accuracy (or concordance) in studies comparing this modality with glass slides. Some newer WSI scanners now incorporate functionality to allow users to remotely control microscope instrument components for real-time robotic telepathology. However, when using the live view mode additional slides often cannot be scanned. The main limitations of WSI include the cost of scanners, the length of time to scan slides, the need for sufficient storage of large digital files, and problems with resolution or fine focusing. Some WSI scanners are capable of producing Z-stack (multiple vertical layers) images to help overcome focusing problems. Due to the aforementioned constraints, WSI scanners have been more useful for second opinion teleconsultation than for use during on-site evaluations.

Implementation and Maintenance

Table 16.2 highlights many of the factors that need to be taken into consideration when implementing and maintaining a telepathology system. Several attributes to this process

TABLE 16.2 Practical considerations regarding telepathology (modified from Pantanowitz et al. J Pathol Inform. 2012;3:45)

Cost	Direct (hardware, software) and indirect (staff, digital file storage)
Distance	Time zones and downtime (cytopathologist should be close enough to be on-site for equipment failure)
Education	Clinician expectations and user training
Networks	Bandwidth limitation, firewalls and security
Computers	Compatibility with enterprise systems
Maintenance	Timely vendor support, IT staff and clinical availability
Images	Formats (may be proprietary), LIS integration and storage (image retention policy)
Metadata	Access to clinical information ± relevant clinical/imaging or relevant lab data
Workflow	Handling of aspirated material, slides and multiple specimens to be transmitted digitally
Regulations	Validation, QA (e.g., CAP telepathology checklist) and billing
Medicolegal	Credentialing, licensing and malpractice coverage
Human factor	Professional reluctance, training and monitoring performance

CAP College of American Pathologists, *IT* information technology, *LIS* laboratory information system, *QA* quality assurance

are unique to cytopathology. Given that cytological preparations often contain material on the slide (e.g., overlapping cells or three-dimensional clusters) that can be difficult to view in focus with a digital image, particular attention should be paid to employing imaging devices that can acquire high resolution images with possible Z-stacking capability. Since multiple different stains are usually performed in cytology, there may be a larger number of slides to digitize compared to surgical pathology. For these reasons, telecytology validation studies should specifically utilize cytology cases.

Conclusion

Telecytology is being increasingly adopted in the practice of cytopathology. With advances in technology, cytologists have shifted from transmitting static images to using more sophisticated technology such as WSI scanners. Telecytology is suitable for handling remote on-site evaluations and for facilitating consultations between distant sites. This results in better utilization of the cytologist's time, facilitates easier access to experts, as well as improvements in the quality and timeliness of patient care. Apart from using a reliable and validated system, it is important to be aware that diagnostic accuracy with telecytology improves with experience and training. Newer telecytology devices will provide better quality digital cytology images that are easier to save, transmit, and navigate for screening and interpretation.

Chapter 17
Cytology Online

Walid E. Khalbuss

Introduction

The Internet has changed how medical information is stored, distributed, and used around the world. In cytopathology, the Internet is increasingly being utilized to aid with clinical work (e.g., Web-based telecytology), eEducation (webinars, online atlases, virtual slide libraries, eJournal), and connectivity among cytologists (e.g., electronic newsletters, Listservs) (Table 17.1). Table 17.2 explains some common terms related to the Internet.

The Internet is a global system of interconnected public and private computer networks linked by wired and wireless technologies. The World Wide Web (WWW) hosts vast amounts of information and provides many services, such as interlinked hypertext documents (Web pages) and e-mail. Many individuals, organizations, businesses (vendors) and

W.E. Khalbuss, M.D., Ph.D., F.I.A.C. (✉)
Department of Pathology, University of Pittsburgh Medical Center
Shadyside, Pittsburgh, PA, USA
e-mail: khalbuss@yahoo.com

L. Pantanowitz and A.V. Parwani (eds.), *Practical Informatics for Cytopathology*, Essentials in Cytopathology 14, DOI 10.1007/978-1-4614-9581-9_17, © Springer Science+Business Media New York 2014

TABLE 17.1 Selected cytology Web sites and links

Web site	URL
CytologyStuff.com	http://www.cytologystuff.com/
Cytopathnet	http://www.cytopathnet.org/tiki-galleries.php
Cytologyweb	http://www.cytologyweb.ch/accueilang.htm
Bethesda System Web Atlas	http://nih.techriver.net/
Cytopathology Image Search	http://137.189.150.85/cytopathology/Slide/CytologyImageSearch.asp
ASC Guidelines Online	http://www.cytopathology.org/website/article.asp?id=2150
IAC Virtual Slide Library	http://www.cytology-iac.org/educational-resources/virtual-slide-library
PSC Thyroid Image Atlas	http://www.papsociety.com/atlas.html
UPMC Case of the Month	http://path.upmc.edu/casemonth.html
JHU Cytopathology Atlas	http://pathology2.jhu.edu/cyto_tutorial/Atlas/

professional societies today have some online presence. Listservs are a great resource for members of cytology organizations that provide a quick way for them to connect with each other, allowing subscribers to the list to receive answers and comments to questions or opinions they may have posted (Fig. 17.1). Use of RSS (Rich Site Summary) allows daily listserv traffic to be condensed into a single Web feed format. Web 2.0 technology offers interactive tools that support social networking (e.g., Facebook) and online sharing (e.g., Google documents).

Online (virtual) education has boomed because of its ability to save time and money, making high-quality cytology education affordable and within reach to cytologists and trainees around the globe. As a result, we have witnessed a transition in cytology practice, education and training away from using traditional tools (e.g., glass teaching slides, textbooks,

TABLE 17.2 Common Internet terms

Term	Explanation
Blog	A discussion or informational Web site that consists of posts
Browser	A software application used to access and present information on the Web (e.g., Internet Explorer, Firefox, Chrome, Safari)
Directory	An organized collection of links to Web sites
Domain	An address for a computer network (e.g., www.cytology.com)
HTTP	Hypertext Transfer Protocol is an application protocol for data communication on the Web
HTML	HyperText Markup Language is the main computer language used for creating Web pages
Hypertext	Text with hyperlinks (links to Web pages)
IP address	An Internet Protocol address is a unique identifying number for each computer on the Internet (e.g., 10.127.0.101)
Listserv	Software that allows a user to send and receive e-mails from a list of subscribers
Search engine	Software used to search for information on the Web (e.g., Google, Bing)
TCP/IP	Protocol (messaging rules) for electronic communication on the Internet
URL	A Uniform Resource Locator is a Web address (e.g., http://cytology)
Web 2.0	Interactive second-generation Web tools that allow users to collaborate and share information online
Web site	A set of related Web pages served from a single Web domain

didactic lectures) to more accessible online resources (e.g., digital slides, Web sites, teleconferences). Combined with advances in digital imaging, particularly whole slide imaging (WSI) technology, the Internet has ushered in tools that further enhance education and practice. For example, offering

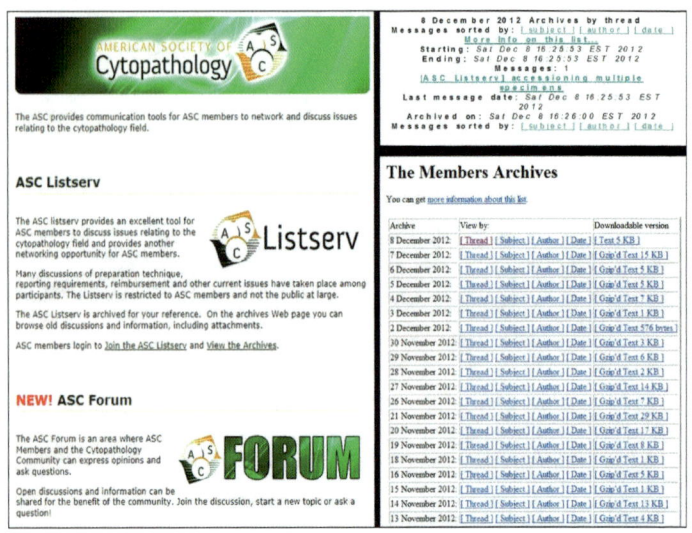

FIG. 17.1 Listserv discussions (called threads) of the American Society of Cytopathology (ASC) are archived and searchable to members

WSI cases online ahead of conferences greatly diminishes the logistics and cost associated with manually mailing glass slides to participants. These tools have created great opportunities in cytopathology for online (virtual) training, education, self assessment, proficiency testing, and research.

Cytology Web sites

There are several educational online cytology Web sites. These Web sites may include static digital images (e.g., NCI Bethesda System Web Atlas), WSI technology (e.g., USCAP Slide Box), audio media (e.g., recorded lectures and seminars), as well as videos (e.g., video of FNA technique on the Papanicolaou Society for Cytopathology Web site). Their educational content is designed to be interactive, often in the

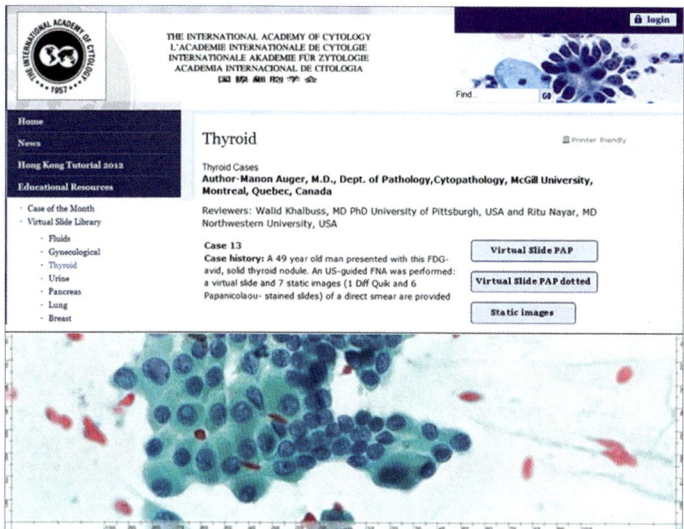

FIG. 17.2 An online cytology teaching case is shown in the Virtual Slide Library on the Web site of the International Academy of Cytology (IAC). Note that the user has a choice to select virtual slides (*unmarked* or *dotted*) or static images of this case

form of a Case of the Month or Virtual Slide Library (Fig. 17.2). WSI allows visitors to a Web site to review the entire digital slide, which simulates traditional light microscopy. These educational Web sites, typically created by academic institutions and professional societies, provide cost-effective training and continuing medical education (CME) opportunities to an international audience. For many years the College of American Pathologists (CAP) mailed cytologists reference glass slides through their Interlaboratory Comparison Program. This educational program allowed participants to assess their screening and interpretive skills. However, these programs were unable to deliver multiple slides of rare and unusual cases. To overcome this limitation, the CAP now offers this educational program online using WSI technology.

Teleconferences and Webinars

The Internet permits cytology educational material to be delivered remotely to multiple individuals in different locations using teleconferences and webinars (Fig. 17.3). A teleconference or webinar is a live exchange of online educational material. An example of such an e-Educational activity is the American Society of Cytopathology (ASC) Cytoeconferences. Audiovisual equipment (e.g., webcams) and software solutions (e.g., GoToMeeting, Skype, Vidyo, WebEx) have become affordable (Fig. 17.3). The host/presenter typically shares their computer desktop which shows up on the screen of all participants who log into the online conference room. The host can show their PowerPoint slides, view virtual slides, or share any other application from their

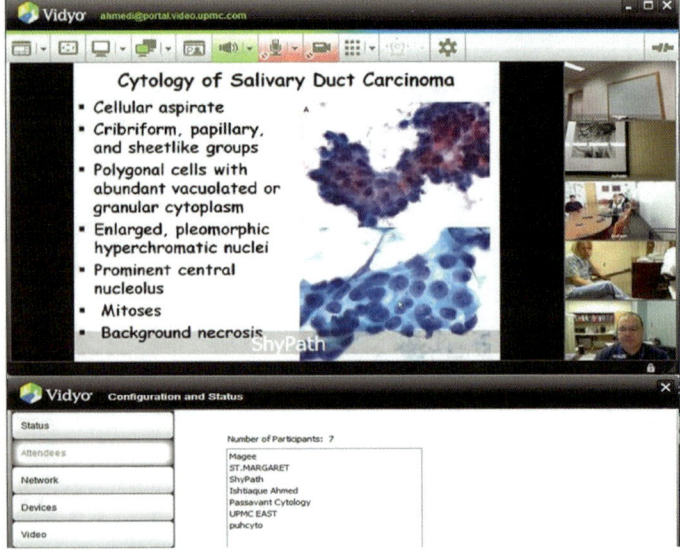

FIG. 17.3 This teleconference on salivary glands was broadcast in real-time via the Internet to seven different medical centers using Vidyo software

desktop. Sessions can be recorded and archived for future use. Software used with these online sessions can allow hosts to track the number of attendees that have signed up, employ interactive techniques such as audience polling, and allow attendees to ask questions in real-time (e.g., "raise a hand" tool).

Online Publications

There are few freely available online journals (e.g., Cytojournal) and publications (e.g., ASC Bulletin, Papanicolaou Society for Cytopathology Focus Newsletter) that deal primarily with cytopathology. Most other subscription cytology journals offer their readers print and online versions. Open access publications provide users unrestricted online access to peer-reviewed scholarly articles. It is anticipated that cytology journals will soon begin to incorporate more interactive technology (e.g., WSI linked to articles).

Chapter 18
Bioinformatics

Somak Roy, Liron Pantanowitz, and Anil V. Parwani

Introduction

Bioinformatics is the discipline of science that deals with the application of mathematics, statistics, and computational methods for processing genomic information which may include, but are not limited to, DNA/RNA sequences, protein sequences, nucleic acid and protein structure, gene expression data, functional annotation, signaling pathways, as well as genotype-phenotype and genotype-therapeutic correlation. Bioinformatics also involves the design and maintenance of large-scale molecular databases, algorithm pipeline development for automating genomic workflow, use of information systems, web technology, imaging, mathematical modeling and computer simulation. Although there is a wide repertoire

S. Roy, M.D. (✉) • L. Pantanowitz, M.D.
A.V. Parwani, M.D., Ph.D., M.B.A.
Department of Pathology, University of Pittsburgh Medical Center,
Pittsburgh, PA, USA
e-mail: roysomak4@gmail.com; pantanowitzl@upmc.edu;
parwaniav@upmc.edu

L. Pantanowitz and A.V. Parwani (eds.), *Practical Informatics*   175
for Cytopathology, Essentials in Cytopathology 14,
DOI 10.1007/978-1-4614-9581-9_18,
© Springer Science+Business Media New York 2014

of bioinformatics applications in biological research, the exponential growth of genomic medicine, introduction of personalized health care, public availability of genomic data, and privacy of health information have made bioinformatics one of the most visible fields in modern science.

The era of molecular diagnostics and targeted therapy has placed increasing demands on cytopathologists to provide adequate cytologic material for diagnostic, prognostic, and research purposes. Cytology offers an excellent means to procure highly diagnostic samples in a minimally invasive way. As little as a few hundred cells can yield enough genetic material to perform high-throughput molecular analyses. The results of such analyses, in turn, may have a profound impact on patient management, as well as fuel innovative research in biomarker discovery and new drug development. Therefore, it is important that cytologists are familiar with bioinformatics and its applications.

Background

The field of bioinformatics emerged from a conglomeration of mathematics, algorithm design, computational science and biology. Mathematical modeling used to predict protein and nucleic acid structure began in the 1950s. One of the best early examples of this field is Watson and Crick's work on unraveling the structure of DNA and "cracking" the genetic code. Paulien Hogeweg coined the term "bioinformatics" in 1978. Subsequent progress in genomics and computer technology permitted the field of bioinformatics to grow exponentially. Prior to 2000, bioinformatics endeavors served largely to support systems used to analyze and manage voluminous genomic data. However, with the advent of high throughput technologies (e.g., microarray gene expression profiling, massive parallel sequencing), unique datasets and bioinformatics challenges emerged that transformed the practice of bioinformatics into an independent field.

Significant advances that helped shape this field included the storage of laboratory data in centrally managed, publically available genomic databases (e.g., GenBank, EMBL data library) and the development of open source software (e.g., BioPerl, BioJava, Integrated Genome Viewer, SHRiMP, Galaxy, and Atlas2).

Computational Requirements

Bioinformatics applications today need to handle large and complex molecular and digital image data. High throughput data generated by high-density microarray chips and next generation sequencers demand large-scale hardware support to process such data in a reasonable amount of time. For example, to analyze and report the sequence variation of a targeted area that covers only a tiny fraction of the entire human genome, a dedicated server is required with plenty of computer processing capability (e.g., at least two 4–6 core processors with 32–48 gigabytes of RAM) and hard disk space (e.g., 8–12 terabytes). Dedicated network connections with high bandwidth are also needed, especially when data needs to be backed up off site. With whole exome and whole genome sequencing, system requirements scale up exponentially, and typically require cluster computing or supercomputers to handle the magnitude of data generated. Even with these information technology resources, however, the processing time for such analyses may take several hours to days to perform. The creation and maintenance of large publically available databases require tremendous infrastructure. These databases are usually hosted in datacenters with many dedicated servers and connectivity with large bandwidth to sustain uninterrupted user access. Such datacenters need to hire not only dedicated bioinformaticists, but often also statisticians, systems analysts, data managers, web programmers, and network support personnel to maintain their infrastructure.

Applications

The scope of bioinformatics is wide. Most applications can be broadly classified into genomic sequence analysis, genomic databases, and related information management, as well as protein structure and function analysis.

Genomic Sequence Analysis

One of the major applications of bioinformatics has been to unravel known and novel sequence variations of the human genome. The advent of targeted therapy, which relies heavily on the mutation profile of tumors, has brought bioinformatics into the limelight. A basic sequencing experiment (e.g., using traditional Sanger sequencing technology) yields a result (or read) comprising a variable containing 100–600 nucleotide bases. Each nucleotide base is assigned a statistical probability score (Phred™ score). The read is then aligned to the reference sequence (called alignment) by software algorithms. Any variation from the reference is detected as a sequence variant (SV) (referred to as variant calling). The detected SV is then annotated manually by pathologists or automatically using a set of algorithms based on public molecular databases and existing literature. With next generation sequencing (NGS), the output generates a massive flat file that consists of millions of reads, where each read is represented by a string of 100–300 nucleotide bases. Processing this amount of data involves significant computational power as well as more redundancy and error checking to establish high statistical confidence in detecting sequence variation.

Genomic Databases

Efficient storage, indexing and distribution of massive amounts of genomic data are an integral part of bioinformatics. Typically, the results of a simple sequence analysis experiment are stored in a flat file. However, storage and indexing of very large-scale information (millions to billions of records) is impractical using the flat file format. This is largely because flat files do not allow for efficient query of stored data. Relational databases are better for these purposes (e.g., MySQL, Microsoft SQL Server, Microsoft Access, Oracle). They have permitted large knowledge databases to be created (e.g., Ensemble genome browser, NCBI genome and variant databases, 1,000 genomes project, Catalogue of Somatic Mutations in Cancer or COSMIC) that house detailed structural, demographic, and clinicopathologic information about many genes, proteins, and sequence variants. They also include reference to relevant literature and links to other databases.

Proteomics

The proteome refers to the entire complement of proteins. Proteomics is the large-scale study of the structure and function of these proteins. The field of proteomics also includes

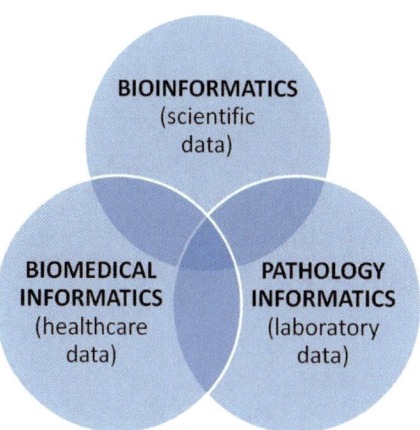

FIG. 18.1 Relationship between bioinformatics, biomedical informatics, and pathology (clinical) informatics

protein purification experiments and mass spectrometry. Like genomics, proteomics generates large datasets which require significant computational support for meaningful interpretation.

Biomedical Informatics

Traditionally, bioinformatics and biomedical informatics were separate components of informatics (Fig. 18.1). Biomedical informatics deals specifically with processing and managing health-related (clinical) data. However, with emerging molecular trends in medicine the overlap among these informatics disciplines has broadened. The use of bioinformatics technology to support clinical testing, and laboratory information systems as a source of so-called "Big Data" for research, are examples where the distinction between these fields is becoming ever more blurred.

Chapter 19
Research Informatics

Somak Roy, Liron Pantanowitz, and Anil V. Parwani

Introduction

Research plays a critical role in the progressive improvement of cytopathology diagnostics and its clinical application. Hence, cytologists need to be aware of the essential informatics issues related to conducting research. This is particularly the case where advances in technology (e.g., computerized databases, the Internet, genetic testing) have opened the door to potential, unintentional breaches of private/confidential health information. Privacy concerns people (e.g., investigators who access information from patients), whereas confidentiality concerns data (e.g., how researchers handle and disseminate identifiable private information). Research in pathology predominantly involves the use of human samples derived from diagnostic specimens (e.g., FNA procedures), as

S. Roy, M.D. (✉) • L. Pantanowitz, M.D.
A.V. Parwani, M.D., Ph.D., M.B.A.
Department of Pathology, University of Pittsburgh Medical Center,
Pittsburgh, PA, USA
e-mail: roysomak4@gmail.com; pantanowitzl@upmc.edu;
parwaniav@upmc.edu

L. Pantanowitz and A.V. Parwani (eds.), *Practical Informatics for Cytopathology*, Essentials in Cytopathology 14,
DOI 10.1007/978-1-4614-9581-9_19,
© Springer Science+Business Media New York 2014

well as pathology data (e.g., cytology reports, ancillary test results). Large-scale research often requires an organized biorepository of various samples (e.g., tissue, serum, isolated DNA), frequently referred to as tissue banks. The principal function of a tissue bank is to store specimens in various forms (e.g., frozen, formalin-fixed paraffin-embedded or FFPE) along with relevant clinical annotations. Since clinical details often contain patient information (e.g., demographics, surgical procedures, laboratory values, survival data), they may act as potential identifiers that endanger misuse of confidential health information. In order to secure protected health information (PHI) in the USA, the Health Insurance Portability and Accountability Act (HIPAA) was initiated in 1996. HIPAA helps define de-identification (temporarily stripping data of identifiable information, but enabling re-linking by a trusted party) and anonymization (irreversibly severing data from any identity) of data. Handling of patient information in a secure manner is the responsibility of the researcher, their affiliated institution, as well as the personnel directly involved in handling such data.

Tissue Banking

Tissue banks provide an invaluable resource of biological specimens for conducting research. Pathologists are often the custodians of these biorepositories. The role of the tissue bank is not only to archive banked samples but also to handle the clinical annotation associated with these specimens. Information technology (IT) required to run a tissue bank includes computers and software necessary to support large and secure relational databases, specimen tracking, inventory management, Web-based applications for users to perform queries, algorithms for encrypting and de-identifying data to secure PHI, and networks that facilitate safe sharing of data across multiple sites. Informatics staff will need to be involved with setting up and maintaining interfaces that permit data to be extracted from disparate information systems to be transmitted and housed in the tissue bank's electronic database. Working with discrete data elements in a format with standardized annotation is extremely important to promote interoperability and the ability to easily share information among researchers.

Protected Health Information

An inherent risk in conducting biomedical research is the potential unauthorized disclosure of patient data leading to a breach in patient confidentiality and privacy. HIPAA regulations help ensure security of PHI for both clinical practice and research. However, biomedical research must also follow institutional guidelines and ethical codes. Research projects therefore typically require Institutional Review Board (IRB) approval. The IRB is a committee whose primary function is to safeguard the rights and welfare of research subjects by critically reviewing research protocols for potential issues related to the use of PHI, ethics and scientific conduct. For most clinical cytology research projects an IRB approval includes a waiver to obtain consent from each individual research subject participating in the study. Depending on the nature of the research (e.g., clinical trials), however, informed consent from all individuals may be mandatory. A research project may solicit the help of an honest broker. This is a designated person not directly involved with the study whose primary function is to obtain clinical data for the researcher, and de-identify or anonymize it by creating indirect identifiers. Several algorithms and protocols exist for de-identifying or anonymizing PHI. Some of the techniques used include time shifting (creating new dates by maintaining constant relative time gaps), substractive data scrubbing, concept map data scrubbing, age range substitution, doublet parsing, using nonunique datasets, and 1-way hashing algorithms (hash values linking to patient encounter). Typical data points that have been recognized as potential identifiers for PHI include names, geographic location, dates, postal address, telephone and fax numbers, social security number, medical record number, a computer's Internet Protocol (IP) address, vehicle registration number, and full face photographs. Finally, it is important to be aware of the consequences related to the improper use of PHI. Penalties under HIPAA regulations are both civil and criminal, depending on the nature of the offense. Violations may lead to imposition of penalties on the institution as well as the researcher. This may involve the suspension of research activities, loss of research funding, monetary fines (e.g., up to $1,500,000/year), and imprisonment (e.g., for up to 10 years).

Appendix A: Key Definitions

Admission, Discharge and Transfer (ADT) ADT systems are software systems used by healthcare facilities to track patients from arrival through to departure. ADT feeds transmit patient demographics to the LIS.

Application software This software causes the computer to perform tasks. On the "front end" (user view) laboratory staff interact with this layer of the LIS by using built-in user interfaces. On the "back end" (administrative view) the LIS application software interacts with the DBMS or with computer/network hardware to communicate the user's commands.

Authentication This is the process of confirming the identity of a person who is attempting to access a system or of confirming the authenticity of a message.

Bandwidth This is the amount of data that can be transmitted via a telecommunication channel from one point to another in a given time period. It is usually expressed in bits (of data) per second (bps).

Binary A numeric system that uses only two digits. All computers operate in binary, or base-2. In other words, all values are stored as (and all calculations are performed in) zeroes and ones.

L. Pantanowitz and A.V. Parwani (eds.), *Practical Informatics for Cytopathology*, Essentials in Cytopathology 14, DOI 10.1007/978-1-4614-9581-9, © Springer Science+Business Media New York 2014

Bioinformatics Bioinformatics is the discipline of science that deals with the application of mathematics, statistics, and computational methods for processing genomic information which may include, but are not limited to, DNA/RNA sequences, protein sequences, nucleic acid and protein structure, gene expression data, functional annotation, signaling pathways, as well as genotype–phenotype and genotype–therapeutic correlation.

Biomedical informatics This branch of informatics deals specifically with processing and managing health-related (clinical) data.

Central Processing Unit (CPU) The CPU is considered to be the "brains" of a computer, performing all logical and derived arithmetic operations on binary data. An example is the Intel core microprocessor.

Change control A process that ensures that changes are recorded, evaluated, authorized and monitored in a controlled and coordinated fashion. This applies to any changes (revisions, alterations, additions, enhancements or upgrades) performed on hardware or software. These changes may be required by a vendor, IT services or by the laboratory.

Charged Coupled Device (CCD) Light entering a camera lens passes through a sensor called a CCD that converts light into a digital image. The resolution of a digital camera is often limited by this image sensor.

Client–server A networking architecture model where client systems (workstations) communicate over a network with server systems. This type of LIS architecture is commonly used by laboratories today. Applications that perform tasks get distributed between the servers (computer hosts that provide a resource or service) and clients (computers that request a service, but do not share their resources).

Clinical Decision Support System (CDSS) Clinical Decision Support (CDS) tools are rule-based or artificial intelligence-based systems that attempt to utilize decision-making science techniques to assist users in making better decisions.

Cloud computing Cloud computing is used to describe a scenario in which user programs and user data are stored online on distributed servers, to be accessed either via a Web browser or via an installable application with access to the Internet. It offers end-users computation, software, data access and storage services without requiring knowledge of the physical location and configuration of the system that delivers such services.

Computerized Provider Order Entry (CPOE) CPOE (also sometimes referred to as computerized physician order entry) enables physicians and other qualified providers to place orders electronically, instead of by paper or telephone. CPOE can be used not only for laboratory tests, but also for ordering medications and other tests (e.g. radiology imaging).

Cookie A minute piece of information that is stored as a text file on your computer that a Web server will use when you browse certain Web sites that you have visited before. Cookies are commonly used when you sign up for services or for sign in features.

Current Procedural Terminology (CPT) A code set listing medical procedures and services performed by healthcare providers, utilized in electronic billing transactions.

Data mining This refers to the act of having a computer that automatically analyzes large quantities of data to identify meaningful, statistically significant patterns.

Databases These are organized collections of digital data. They are created and manipulated by programs known as database management systems (DBMS), many of which are designed for very specific purposes (e.g. Microsoft Excel, Microsoft Access, MySQL, Oracle).

Database Management System (DBMS) This refers to a specialized software that helps control the access, organization, storage, management, querying and retrieval of data from databases.

Deming cycle This cycle is also known as the PDCA (plan–do–check–act) cycle. This four-step management method is used for the control and continuous improvement of many processes and products.

Dictionaries Dictionaries are tables, sometimes also called maintenance files. They are components of the LIS database that play a significant role in defining data formats, structures, and rules. Examples include tables containing lists of physician names, special stains, diagnoses used for reporting (e.g. The Bethesda System terminology), billing codes, users passwords and so on.

Digital Imaging and Communications in Medicine (DICOM) This is a standard used for medical imaging. DICOM is the universal format used to primarily handle images in the radiology Picture Archiving and Communication System (PACS).

Disaster recovery This refers to a set of processes, policies and procedures that can enable recovery and continuation of critical IT infrastructure after a disaster. Disasters may be natural (e.g. floods, fire) or human-related (e.g. power failure, hacker, hazardous chemical spill, bioterrorism). A disaster recovery plan is also referred to as a "business continuity plan".

Electronic Health Record (EHR) The EHR, also known as an electronic medical record (EMR), is a patient's medical chart that can be accessed and modified in digital format.

Encryption This is the activity of converting data or information into code that can be applied to text messages or other important data, so that it is altered to make it humanly unreadable (except by someone who knows how to decrypt it).

Extensible Markup Language (XML) A hierarchical markup language that allows for documents to be encoded in machine-readable form. XML was created to structure, store and transport information.

Firewall This is a network security system comprised of software or hardware intended to control incoming and outgoing network traffic.

Firmware This is software installed on a memory chip on a hardware device (e.g. the software program pre-installed on a digital camera or flash drive).

Graphics Processing Unit (GPU) This unit serves to create images that are displayed on a monitor, which may sometimes also be used for general-purpose and computing 3D calculations.

Grid computing This is conceptually similar to cloud computing, except that in grid computing the servers are usually owned by or under the authority of the end user. Grid computing is most often used to bind together many different computer systems, allowing them to function as a virtual "supercomputer".

Hard drive A hard disk drive is a high-capacity, self-contained storage device that contains a read–write mechanism, as well as one or more hard disks located inside a sealed unit.

Hardware This refers to the mechanical components of the computer and includes the central processing unit (CPU), motherboard, volatile storage, graphical processing unit (GPU), input devices such as the keyboard and mouse, output devices such as monitors and speakers, as well as other peripheral devices.

Health Information Exchange (HIE) This refers to the transmission of healthcare information electronically across organizations—not only within hospital systems but also across large regions.

Health Level 7 (HL7) This is the most commonly employed interchange standard that defines how electronic messages are transmitted between electronic health records. HL7 provides a set of rules that permit data to be shared and processed by healthcare organizations in a uniform and consistent manner.

Informatics This is the science of information that involves storing, processing, accessing and communicating information, leading to the conversion of data into information to solve complex problems.

Information Technology (IT) This refers more to the technical aspects of this field related to computers, telecommunications (networking) and digital imaging equipment.

Interface Interfaces are bridges between computer hardware, peripheral devices or information systems. An interface between an EHR and another piece of software is called an application interface; instrument interfaces are the links between an EHR and hardware instruments; and user interfaces are the text and graphical elements by which human beings interact with the EHR.

Interface engine A program that integrates and centralizes many different application interfaces. They allow different computer systems to access and exchange information.

International Classification of Diseases (ICD) A standard healthcare classification of diagnostic codes used for epidemiology, health management and clinical purposes.

Laboratory Information System (LIS) A large, complex system made up of software and hardware that handles electronic data to support laboratory operations.

Logical Observations Identifiers and Codes (LOINC) A dataset and universal code system for identifying medical laboratory observations.

Mainframe This refers to a large, high-speed, room-spanning computer that supports numerous workstations or peripherals.

Malware A program that has a harmful effect (intentional or unintentional) on a computer's operating system, other user programs, or user data. Computer viruses and spyware fall into this category of software.

Meaningful use This refers to the use of certified electronic health record (EHR) technology by providers in ways that can be measured significantly in quality and in quantity.

Middleware Hardware and/or software inserted between lab instruments and the LIS. Middleware connects a legacy LIS to newer systems in order to add functionality.

Motherboard This is the unit inside a computer upon which all other components are mounted and electrically connected.

Network This is a group of two or more computer systems that are linked together.

Ontology A vocabulary that includes information about the relationships between concepts; this allows for an under-standing of the structure of the information, and facilitates advanced information processing.

Operating system (OS) This is the central piece of software through which the capabilities of a computer can be operated. Common operating systems include Microsoft Windows, Mac OS, Linux, Android and iOS.

Picture Archive and Communications system (PACS) A collec-tion of medical imaging technology systems, servers and work-stations used for storage, rapid retrieval, and widespread access to mainly digital radiology images.

Pixel A digital image is composed of thousands of tiny pixels (PIcture ELements) regularly arranged in rows and columns. Pixels are rectangular shaped. Each pixel contains data (binary 0 and 1), storing values such as brightness and color.

Protected Health Information (PHI) This refers to any infor-mation related to healthcare that can be linked to a specific individual. According to HIPAA in the USA, there are 18 identifiers that may link an individual to PHI (e.g. medical record number, zip code, etc.).

Radio-Frequency Identification (RFID) RFID tags are small transponders that use radio frequency signals. When affixed to an asset they can store unique data about that asset. There are both active and passive RFID tags.

Regional Health Information Organizations (RHIOs) These are a group of organizations with a business stake in trying to integrate and exchange healthcare information with all mem-bers of the healthcare community (hospitals, medical societ-ies, payers and employers).

Request for information (RFI) A request addressed to a potential vendor to inquire about products and services available.

Request for price quotation (RPQ) A document used to solicit vendor price quotations based on major requirements and operational statistics.

Request for proposal (RFP) An invitation for vendors to submit a detailed proposal on their product/service in response to specific stated requirements.

Resolution Image resolution refers to the amount of detail that a digital image holds; i.e. the pixel count for each dimension of the image (resolution = image width × height; measured in pixels). Display resolution refers to the level of information on a computer display.

Server A high-powered computational platform that can be mounted on standardized frameworks known as racks, either horizontally or vertically.

Six Sigma Six Sigma is based on the concept that defects (errors) and variability in processes (manufacturing) can be reduced by effectively using data and statistical analysis. The ideal goal is to fix a process so that it will be 99.9997 % defect free (six Standard Deviations) or produce only 3.4 defects per million opportunities (DPMO).

Systematized Nomenclature of Medicine (SNOMED) A collection of medical terms that provides a consistent way to index, store, retrieve, and aggregate medical data across specialties and sites of care.

Structured Query Language (SQL) This is a standard computer language commonly used to access data stored in databases.

Telecytology This refers to the remote transmission of digital cytology images for evaluation at a distance.

Toyota Production System (TPS) The TPS, developed by Toyota for their automobile manufacturing, refers to a management philosophy and practices that are directed towards organizing manufacturing and logistics, including the interaction with suppliers and customers.

Unified Medical Language System (UMLS) This is a comprehensive list of biomedical terms used for developing computer systems that are capable of understanding the specialized vocabulary used in biomedicine and healthcare.

Whole slide imaging (WSI) This refers to the digitization of an entire glass slide with a scanner in order to generate a digital (virtual) slide (i.e. whole slide image).

Workstation These are high-powered computational platforms connected to a network, geared toward the act of content creation.

Z-axis This refers to the vertical axis in a three-dimensional Cartesian coordinate system. Certain WSI scanners are able to digitize a glass slide along multiple z-axis planes (z stacking).

Appendix B: Recommended Reading

Textbooks

Pantanowitz L, Balis UJ, Tuthill JM. Pathology informatics: theory & practice. Chicago: ASCP Press; 2012.

Articles

Becich MJ, Gilbertson JR, Gupta D, Patel A, Grzybicki DM, Raab SS. Pathology and patient safety: the critical role of pathology informatics in error reduction and quality initiatives. Clin Lab Med. 2004; 24(4):913–43.

Cucoranu IC, Parwani AV, West AJ, Romero-Lauro G, Nauman K, Carter AB, Balis UJ, Tuthill MJ, Pantanowitz L. Privacy and security of patient data in the pathology laboratory. J Pathol Inform. 2013;4:4.

Henricks WH. "Meaningful use" of electronic health records and its relevance to laboratories and pathologists. J Pathol Inform. 2012;3:39.

Khalbuss WE, Pantanowitz L, Parwani AV. Digital imaging in cytopathology. Pathology Research International. 2011; Article ID 264683.

Pantanowitz L, Henricks WH, Beckwith BA. Medical laboratory informatics. Clin Lab Med. 2007;27:823–43.

Pantanowitz L, Hornish M, Goulart RA. Informatics applied to cytology. Cytojournal. 2008;5:16.

Pantanowitz L, Hornish M, Goulart RA. The impact of digital imaging in the field of cytopathology. Cytojournal. 2009;6:6.

Park S, Pantanowitz L, Sharma G, Parwani AV. Anatomic pathology laboratory information systems: a review. Adv Anat Pathol. 2012a;19: 81–96.

Park S, Pantanowitz L, Parwani AV. Digital imaging in pathology. Clin Lab Med. 2012b;32:557–84.

Park S, Parwani A, Aller RD, Banach L, Becich MJ, Borkenfeld S, Carter AB, Friedman BA, Rojo MG, Georgiou A, Kayser G, Kayser K, Legg M, Naugler C, Sawai T, Weiner H, Winsten D, Pantanowitz L. The history of pathology informatics: a global perspective. J Pathol Inform. 2013;4:7.

Thrall M, Pantanowitz L, Khalbuss WE. Telecytology: clinical applications, current challenges and future benefits. J Pathol Inform. 2011;2:51.

Wilbur DC. Digital cytology: current state of the art and prospects for the future. Acta Cytol. 2011;55(3):227–38.

Williams S, Henricks WH, Becich MJ, Toscano M, Carter AB. Telepathology for patient care: what am I getting myself into? Adv Anat Pathol. 2010;17(2):130–49.

Index

A
Administrative Simplification provisions, 66
Admission, discharge and transfer (ADT), 20, 55
Altosoft, 87
American Medical Association (AMA), 39
American Recovery and Reinvestment Act (ARRA), 126
Application service provider (ASP) model, 48
Association of Pathology Informatics (API), 2
Atomicity, consistency, isolation, and durability (ACID), 26
Atypical cells of undetermined significance (ASCUS), 81
Automated Pap tests
  autostainers, 147
  cell collection, 147
  cost-effective, 150
  diagnosis, 150
  digital imaging technology accession identification (ID), 150
  BD FocalPoint review station, 151–153
  image processor controller, 150, 151
  imaging station/slide profiler, 150
  slide edge/labels, 151
  ThinPrep review scope, 151–153
  implementation and maintenance, 154–155
  interactive screening systems, 153–154
  LBC, 148–149
  learning curve, 150
  monolayer slide preparation, 147
  primary screening systems, 148–149, 153
  software, 148

B
Barcoding
  1D/2D barcode symbology, 96–97
  hardware
    barcode readers, 100
    cassette printers, 100, 101

L. Pantanowitz and A.V. Parwani (eds.), *Practical Informatics for Cytopathology*, Essentials in Cytopathology 14, DOI 10.1007/978-1-4614-9581-9, © Springer Science+Business Media New York 2014

Printed by Printforce, the Netherlands